M.E., Myself And I

An insider's view of Myalgic Encephalomyelitis & Chronic Fatigue Syndrome

K.C. FINN

ACKNOWLEDGEMENTS

This book is written with copious thanks to my family and friends, for everything they have to put up with, and also to Wendela Poole, without whom I would not have had the courage to put the words on the page.

CONTENTS

Introduction

or

'What is M.E. anyway?'

Have you ever had a powerful impact hit your body? Perhaps you've been clipped by a fast car, been tackled by someone twice your size whilst playing sports, or simply been crashed into by a heavy figure on a busy street. In that moment of impact, several things happen. Your head spins from the shock of the contact. Every nerve in your body buzzes with a sudden wave of pain and discomfort. The area where the impact actually happens hurts so sharply that it makes you want to shout out in agony. Seconds after the moment, your body stings and your blood pressure rises, upsetting your whole system, raising your body temperature, making you want to cry. The whole experience leaves you momentarily exhausted, breathless and aching.

Now imagine feeling that every time you get up from a chair. Imagine that wild, painful impact attacking you when you try to take a shower or make a cup of tea. Imagine that agony coming on suddenly and randomly in the middle of night when you're completely still and fast asleep.

That's M.E.

They call it Myalgic Encephalomyelitis; they call it Chronic Fatigue Syndrome. It doesn't matter if you know what they call it. It matters that you understand what it does to people all around the world. What it does to people like me.

The condition is an invisible disability with no known cure that can attack anyone at any age with no hope of prevention or cure. M.E. affects every major system in your body from your temperature control to your breathing, brain activity, appetite, muscles, nerves and joints. It is a condition that can bring a happy, healthy life to an immediate grinding halt. Some people have it in recurring bouts and some people live with its multitude of nasty symptoms every single day of their lives.

This book is designed to give you an inside look at what the thoughts and feelings of living with M.E. really are. It is split into sections which focus on various aspects of life with the condition, ranging from symptoms to treatments to social and emotional factors. There are plenty of medical books out there to tell you all about the condition and suggest ways in which it can be treated. That's not the purpose of the words you're holding right now. This book is my shoulder to cry on: my way to let fellow sufferers know that they are not alone and to allow those closest to them to step into the world of M.E. and realise what it is we sufferers have to deal with every day.

It is my hope that within these pages there is some capacity for people to gain understanding, to see beyond the illusion of this debilitating condition into its stark realities. It is not a book of stringent advice, because anyone with M.E. will tell you it works differently for every individual concerned. It is not a book that advocates any particular treatment or method of symptom management. It is simply a frank discussion of how my illness makes me feel and what it has taught me, delivered here in the hope that this message can, in turn, help others take steps towards their own realisations.

So who am I, you might ask, to write such a book? What qualifications do I have that entitle me to print these words about M.E. and its terrorising attacks?

The answer is none at all.

I was thirteen when the condition struck me down. It began with migraine headaches, muscle pains and extreme fatigue. As I was in my teenage years, these symptoms were put down to 'growing pains' and academic pressure. I bounced back and forth to the doctor's for a year to be told there was nothing for my parents to worry about. I stopped talking about my symptoms because I was sick of going to the doctor. I had already decided, in my young mind, what was wrong with me. I was weak, unfit, a little overweight. I just wasn't as good at physical things as other kids. I accepted my reality as a weakling and carried it with me for the next few years.

I was reaching the end of high school when my symptoms worsened yet again, my memory and concentration throwing me off-balance. I started to need to sleep during the day, coming home and collapsing, still in my school uniform, for the hours between the end of the school day and the start of my evening meal. I began to lie awake at night, plagued by anxiety and wild panic attacks with no discernable cause. Unfortunately my parents' break up happened at exactly the same time, so when I returned to the doctors about my sleeplessness, I was misdiagnosed as clinically depressed because of the family split.

I spent the next three years believing that diagnosis outright, expecting that one day I would suddenly be happy again and my tiredness, aching bones, headaches and disturbed sleep would all just disappear when that day came. It was the week of my eighteenth birthday when I realised something very important. I wasn't sad anymore. But I was still sick. I stopped taking all the medication I'd be given by my doctors to convince myself that the 'depression' I'd suffered from was gone, but none of my physical ailments went away, even though my life was pretty good and looking better all the time.

I started pursuing a diagnosis at age nineteen when my symptoms extended to fevers, sweats, stomach problems, blood pressure issues and numbing in my nerves. I was twenty-two before the appropriate tests were finally given, after exhausting several doctors with my pleas and changing surgeries to find a GP who would be willing to help me. By the time the precious letters 'M.E.' came to be written on an official piece of paper, I already knew this was the name of the monster that had haunted for almost half my life. I was pleased to put a name to it, even though it was a sentence I knew I couldn't escape.

I am now twenty-five years old, coming up to twelve years living with this crippling condition. I am a fiction writer, a novelist, living in worlds where daring characters do incredible things and magic and science fiction mean that illnesses like mine can be cured. The prospect of writing about my condition has frightened me for many years, but recently I have come to the conclusion that suffering in silence isn't the right thing to do, no more than it was when I thought I was a weak little girl at school.

If people like me don't speak up, how will anyone ever know how it really feels to live with M.E.? If no-one knows how important it is to promote research and awareness for sufferers, then countless other children will keep their mouths shut when they feel more tired and weak than those around them. They too will spend years feeling like every ounce of pain and every loss of strength is their fault.

This book opens the door to my thoughts and feelings. It's not always pretty and it's not always pleasant, but it is honest, and it comes from a place of hope.

How I Feel Right Now

or

'Nobody can possibly feel that many things at once'

I once knew a civil servant who dealt with disability claims for people with M.E.. "Oh, they put down absolutely *everything*," said she, "they have absolutely *everything* wrong with them." It's not worth trying to challenge that kind of ignorance here and now (although it is both worrying and unsurprising to find those kinds of attitudes in positions of power), but I thought I would try to explain to people outside of the M.E. world exactly what it feels like to have this condition. Fellow sufferers, feel free to nod your heads along as you read this. Non-sufferers, be aware that this is what's happening every day to all the M.E. sufferers that you know.

It's the 6th of March 2014. It's 2:40 in the afternoon. I am twenty-five years old. And this is how I feel right now.

The most noticeable thing is the sharp pain running across the back of my shoulders. This is a constant ache brought on by tension in the surrounding muscles which has been steadily getting worse for a decade. Today the ache is particularly sharp because I am on a new directive to improve my posture and look a little less like the Hunchback of Notre Dame. Every ten minutes or so I sit up straight and put my shoulders into a normal human position instead of the homunculus slouch I usually have while writing. When I do this it feels as though my muscles are stuck together with superglue and I'm trying to stretch them apart. Suffice to say I don't do it for very long and it aches like heck afterwards.

Last night I was suffering from a shooting pain in my left calf that was reminiscent of a trapped nerve or sciatica. Today there's a similar spot just below my left knee at the back of that calf where a very specific ache is throbbing, as though I've been shot in the leg with a paintball. The ache isn't fading. The hysterical woman caged up in the back of my brain is convinced it's a deep vein thrombosis and I'm going to die. I keep her quiet by reminding her that she convinced me I had breast cancer five years ago and I'm still here to tell the tale, so she clearly needs to stop being so crazy.

You know that scene in X-Men 2 where Wolverine injects Lady Deathstrike with loads of liquid metal, and when it dries her head slams down really heavily like a brick? That's what the space at the back of my head is threatening to do right now. It has its own mass that's unrealistically heavy compared to the rest of my body. I feel like if I put my head back on the sofa at this moment, I'm never going to want to lift it up again. Even when I shut my eyes to do my deep breathing and most other things fade away, that heaviness is still there and it seems no amount of pain relief is going to shift it today.

Three fingers of my right hand keep going numb whilst I'm typing. I stop between sentences to roll my wrist and shake them out. I move my arm around to try and be in the right position to promote circulation. I wave like a manic zombie, grateful that the window blinds stop anyone from seeing me do it, but it doesn't go away. The hysterical woman shouts 'DVT! DVT!' again. I carry on typing and hope that it's something that will fix itself when my body decides to work properly again.

I haven't eaten much, so my stomach is convulsing a little. I tried a packet of crisps earlier (low calorie and non-greasy) but the pain of digesting them left me squirming in my seat and I had to get up and walk around until they'd gone down. So now I'm 50% hungry, 50% nauseous and 100% confused about whether to try more food or not. If I do eat something else, I'll have to plan a lie down afterwards whilst I digest, which is going to interrupt my work schedule. On the other hand, dying of starvation isn't on my to-do list either, so maybe a snack and its subsequent fallout will be necessary soon.

My eyes are dry. I don't really have a solution for how to make them un-dry, since water and drops and all that jazz only seems to lead to making them sticky. If sticky and dry are the only two options for my eyeballs, I guess I prefer dry right now, at least it means I can get things done. Of course that also means constant interruptions whilst I stop to rub my eyes in the hope that they'll magically stop being dry. Add to that the habitual motion of repeatedly cleaning my glasses, even though I know the black spots I can see in my vision are actually debris *inside* my eyeballs, not gunk on the lenses.

On top of those irritating things, I'm tired. And it's not like that 'Ooh I'm tired' feeling that normal folk get when they've gone up a flight of stairs a bit too quickly. This is 'I just ran up six flights of stairs whilst carrying a baby elephant' kind of exhaustion. My breath is short and my muscles are burning marathon-recovery style. And what did I do to bring this awful sensation upon myself? I walked about 20 feet to the bathroom and back. Silly me. I should know better than to think that I can walk to the bathroom and not have to pay the price for my transgressions.

So that's how I feel right now. Some of these sensations are pretty much constant and some I resent a lot more than others because they really disturb the few pleasurable things I have in my life. There's one final thing I'd like to put into perspective for you here though:

This is a good day for me.

All these things I'm contending with are completely normal to me and I don't usually go a day without experiencing all of them at some point. If I was having a bad day, I wouldn't be sitting here to write about it, believe me. Unfortunately this is the day-to-day reality of living with M.E.; for some sufferers this reality is even worse. And if you've read this section finding it impossible to believe that one person can be feeling so many things at once, I can only tell you that I sincerely *wish* I was making it up.

K.C. FINN

Fatigue

or

'When they were handing out energy, I was in the bathroom'

I am actively trying not to go back to sleep today. To people outside the understanding of M.E., that's going to sound like a strange statement. Most people resisting the temptation of an afternoon nap are doing so in lieu of a bad night's sleep, a late night out or an incredibly physical, energy-sapping act like a sporting event. Me? I just slept a really good seven and a half hours, but now that I've been awake for four hours my body is starting to fail me. The food I've eaten is a normal amount, but it hasn't been able to provide the sustenance I need to feel slightly less than exhausted. My body is crying out to lie back on the sofa; my eyes are closing on their own even as I type.

Life lived on a flat battery.

It's the best description I have ever heard for how I spend each day of my existence. It's like those last few minutes you get out of your laptop when you know its battery is about to fail; you do everything you can to sustain those last drops of juice. You turn the brightness right down, the sound off, close all unnecessary programs in the background to keep those precious few percentiles of energy going for as long as possible to get your job done. In the end you know it's going to crash, but at least you milked it for all it was worth before you had to give in and charge it up. There's a big problem with doing that though: eventually you're going to give your laptop serious problems by mistreating its battery.

Maybe you can see where I'm going with this already. Running your body down to nothing causes serious problems in healthy people, let alone people who suffer with conditions that bring on chronic fatigue. Any M.E. sufferer will be able to tell you that chronic fatigue is nothing like ordinary tiredness either. Ordinary tiredness goes away with a nice sit down in front of the telly and a cup of tea. Chronic fatigue stays with you, often for several days after what seems like a very minor event. I'm not privy to the official figures on how much longer chronic fatigue lasts than normal tiredness, but from my own experience I know that it usually takes me about three times longer to refresh my energy than those around me when we have all done the same thing. If my best friend and I were to climb a sharp flight of stairs, she might take five minutes to sit and chill afterwards before she could do other things, probably less. I would have to curl up in a perfectly still ball for at least fifteen minutes to even feel remotely human again.

The 'battery' in an M.E. body needs regular

charging to avoid these kinds of problems. If I continue to be active for too long without recuperation, then I'm likely to ruin my whole day (and usually several days after) by trying to burn the candle at both ends. Just because I *can* carry on and use up all my energy doesn't mean I *should*. You may be wondering then, why I said I'm trying not to go back to sleep today. So here's a gem of information that I find invaluable:

Sleep is not the same thing as rest.

For the M.E. sufferer, sleep can be as much of an enemy as it can an ally, especially when it comes to battling against fatigue. Chronic fatigue is *not* caused by a lack of sleep; it's caused by the inability to recover energy properly after exertion, so sleeping isn't necessarily going to make you feel healthy again. In my case, I often wake from an afternoon nap feeling worse than I was before I took it, regretting that I hadn't spent that time doing something more worthwhile. It sounds strange, I know, but restful activities actually top up my energy better than falling asleep.

There are different kinds of things that a body requires energy to do. Some are extremely basic, essential activities such as breathing, temperature control and circulation of the blood. These are the final warning signs in the world of fatigue: if I've run my battery down so badly that it's a struggle to breathe, then unfortunately lying down and being totally immobile tends to be the only option left in order to recover. So the trick is not to let things get that far. Other activities that sap energy include physical movements (even the smallest ones), cognitive tasks (such as reading, writing and having a conversation) and also emotional states which can drain you without you even knowing it (unhappiness is a major energy-sapper). Being aware of what you're using your energy on is the first step to mastering fatigue.

Awareness and balance. Those two words are going to be very familiar to you by the time you're through with this book, I'm sure. For my part, I will tell you honestly that I have not mastered the trick of energy-balancing as yet. I still have days where I fall into the Nap Trap and wake up unhappy that I've wasted two hours of my life kipping without feeling any better for it.

But today, as I said, I am *not* going back to sleep.

Instead, I aim to take appropriate breaks and balance out the different ways I use my energy in order to get things done. It's actually an hour later now than when I started this section of writing (I took some time out to eat and sit quietly with some deep breathing) but having that break has had a definite impact on my ability to continue working. At the start of writing this chapter, I was thinking about switching the laptop off and going for a nap. Now I'm quite happy to start the next chapter, safe in the knowledge that I can stop and recharge, both the machine and myself, whenever I want.

Strength

or

'How kittens beat me in a fight'

I recently wrote a novel for teenagers in which the main character suffers from Juvenile Arthritis. I decided to give this character a physical disability because it made sense to my plot and effectively kept her stuck in one place for the duration of the novel. I chose J.A. because the condition has a lot of musculoskeletal similarities to M.E. and I remember what it was like to be a physically weak teenager with deep-set insecurities. It was easy for me to imagine, convey and relate to that character's struggles as the plot of the novel progressed. They say you should write from what you know, so that's what I tried my hand at with this project.

As it happened, the novel was picked up by a publisher almost as soon as I'd finished writing it. I was excited to see the story championed by these publishers, but once it was time to send the book out for public reviews, I suddenly became concerned about my representation of a disabled young girl. Would readers find the parts of the plot where she struggles with her illness to be boring? Would they even care about her condition or would they simply say she ought to 'get over it' or 'deal with it' as so many people have said to me in years gone by? I became extremely nervous as I awaited the feedback from the first wave of advanced readers in the publishing group. I almost considered pulling the book back out of the deal.

Their reactions were very similar to one another and the general message I got really surprised me. Everyone talked of how strong the main character was. Her struggle and the things that she dealt with every day in the novel were not seen as symbols of inferiority or weakness, but as markers of her strength and courage because of the way she kept on keeping on. One reader referred to it as a silent, hidden strength that people around her didn't even realise she had, but the reader was privy to it because they were inside her head and could feel her pain. I'm not going to lie to you: I cried a little when I read that.

I am in the habit of thinking of myself as weak.

It started years ago, when I first became ill and I didn't know that I had a physical condition. Because I couldn't do the things that other young teens could do, I felt immediately inferior and incompetent in comparison to them. My logical conclusion at the time was that I was a weakling, that I was simply not strong enough to be considered a normal girl. It's a horrible inner belief to grow up with, but it fit with the fact that everything I did hurt and I was constantly tired and unable to do physical activities very well. My parents simply said 'Well, she's just not sporty', as any parent would. None of us knew what was really going on until much later, during my adult life.

My physical capacity for strength is constantly decreasing. A year ago I could still open a milk bottle with little difficulty. Now I don't drink milk until someone comes home to open the plastic cap. I used to be able to lift and drag heavy objects, even if it meant I would suffer extreme fatigue later for doing so. Now I find I can't get most large things like dining chairs off the ground to shift them where I want them to go. It's embarrassing to have to ask for help with everything all the time and my friends and family often catch me struggling to open jars and such with that 'hand it over' look on their faces. That look makes me feel like that young teen weakling all over again, but I have little choice but to accept their help if I want to go on living my life.

The reaction to my novel has helped me to remember that strength can be measured in a variety of different ways. Some of my friends have remarked that they don't know how I manage to go on achieving things such as writing novels when I face so much pain and fatigue every day. They say that they wouldn't have the strength to cope with it like I do. I tend to punish myself for the dark, weak moments when I sit in agony and just want to cry about my illness, but conversely I've realised that I don't reward myself for all those other moments where I just get on with it and do things regardless of the struggle I'm having. I may not be able to open a bottle of milk, but pushing through my considerable pain barrier to even get up in the morning is no mean feat.

If it sounds like I'm ego-boosting, then that's because I am. We're taught to be demure nowadays about achievement, taught that arrogance and pride are deadly sins to be avoided at all costs. This puts a lot of people on the opposite track, leading them to self-doubt and under-confidence in their abilities and prospects. I've been putting myself down for my physical weaknesses for long enough; it's about time I took some pride in my strengths. I spend every day of my life in pain and near-total exhaustion, but I have the strength to do so many things that others take for granted.

I get up in the morning despite the pain. I eat my meals despite the nausea. I get things done despite the fatigue. I face my fears despite the nerves. I crack jokes about my illness despite the sadness of my reality. And I keep going and keep chasing my dreams despite the degenerative prospect of my future.

There are plenty of things that the average person can do that I cannot, but there are also a bucket-load of things I'm capable of that they can't even imagine having to deal with. It's important not to let your weaknesses cast a shadow over your strengths, because just continuing to live with M.E. is a massive achievement in itself, and one that we don't give ourselves enough credit for achieving.

Physical Pain

or

'I feel like Mufasa after the stampede'

One of the reasons why sufferers with this condition prefer the term M.E. over C.F.S. is because the words 'Chronic Fatigue Syndrome' don't really cover all the things that are going on within the patient's body. Fatigue is, undeniably, a huge symptom of the condition, and one which makes all the other parts of the illness even worse. It is also used as a vital part of the diagnostic process. If you don't have crippling, constant fatigue, then you probably don't have M.E., but it doesn't mean that that's the only thing encroaching on your enjoyment of life.

Tiredness brings about pain. We all know this. If you take a flight of stairs too quickly, your legs burn with the strain of it. If you lift something so heavy that it wears you out, you'll feel it in your lungs and muscles for quite a while afterwards. So imagine what it would be like if the amount of effort to run up the stairs was actually the same effort you needed just to lift yourself out of a chair. Imagine if the heavy something you lifted that strained your whole body was only actually as heavy as a milk bottle. I have never been able to carry milk home from the shop (which is 2 minutes from my current home) without having to rest my arms for at least quarter of an hour afterwards because of the intense pain that tiredness and physical strain inflicts on my body.

Something that a lot of people I've known fail to understand is that pain is relative to its sufferer. Two ordinary healthy people can engage in the same activity and one may come away from it aching whilst the other is totally fine. Two people can suffer from the same virus and one may struggle whilst the other is able to continue their normal life in spite of the condition. Pain in the M.E. body is relative to the level of fatigue being inflicted on the sufferer at any given moment. No two days are the same, but every day holds the hidden risk of doing painful damage to oneself through over-exertion, something which the sufferer may not even know they are doing to themselves. If my family see me doing something that looks like a strain, giant red warning sirens go off in their heads and they quickly intervene before the damage can be done.

Physical pain with this condition is also about the nervous system. Because of other tag-along conditions like anxiety and hypersensitivity that we sufferers tend to get, our interpretation of any kind of pain is pretty extreme. I've been known to projectile vomit from the sudden sensation of stubbing my toe. Not a pretty sight, I'll admit, but a valuable warning to look where I'm going in public places in the future. When we react so extremely to what seem like small-pain events, it's not for attention and it's not out of weakness. It's because we live inside bodies that are largely out of our control, constantly reacting to stimuli that most healthy people aren't affected by and wouldn't even recognise as a potential threat to an M.E. sufferer's health.

The blessing of having an invisible disability is that you can hide it easily when you feel all right. The curse is that many people will treat you as weak or abnormal when you're not well because they can't accept the fact that, for example, someone bumping into you on the street can having you crying in agony after the impact has passed (again, a lesson to watch where I'm going and, more importantly, where other people are going, on the street). The most important lesson I have tried to teach my nearest and dearest is to accept the fact that I'm in pain when I tell them so, even if they can't understand the reasons why. Acceptance doesn't make the pain go away, but at least it stops you from feeling worse, like you're not being believed.

The other lesson I can impart here is one for M.E. sufferers themselves and those who might be keeping an eye out for their symptoms:

Any pain that doesn't come from tiredness or injury is **NOT** your M.E. affecting you. Get it checked out.

There was a point in my life where I had accepted that physical pain was a given in anything that I did, day in and day out. Therefore, when waves of pain came around, I accepted them wholeheartedly as part of my lot in life and let them ruin my day, regardless of where they had come from. It took the wise words of a pain specialist to help me see the difference between pain caused by exertion and pain that wasn't supposed to be part of the mix. After that there were some investigations with results that surprised even me.

Arthritis in my jaw and a curvature of the spine were hiding underneath my M.E.

These are both treatable conditions that can be dealt with by doctors to severely reduce pain and improve physical ability, two things that an M.E. sufferer sorely needs in their life. My lack of awareness and despondency in relation to pain meant that I had let both illnesses wreak havoc on my bones and muscles for years without treatment, a mistake which will now take me a very long time to rectify. If I had stopped to analyse my pain instead of pretending it didn't exist, I could have stopped a large proportion of it in its tracks a long time ago.

Physical pain is a horribly unpleasant symptom that feeds into other debilitating parts of M.E. such as emotional pain and depression (both discussed later in this book). Some medications can offer a little help, but ultimately we would all rather not have the pain at all than have to treat it every day. The things that make constant pain a little easier to deal with in my life are knowing what works for me to treat it, through careful analysis, and making sure that those around me are aware that I might suddenly burst into tears if they accidentally stand on my toe.

Hypersensitivity

or

'Stop screaming at me and put that light out'

I was helping to put a sheet on a bed about ten minutes ago and I grazed my leg against the sharp corner of a drawer that was jutting out. It's still aching now, a very small, circular area of pain that feels as though someone has taken a ball-peen hammer and whacked me just once on the bone there. It got me thinking about hypersensitivity, because honestly I barely touched the edge of that drawer, and yet I'm here now trying to type and rub my leg at the same time because the ache there is so intense.

Hypersensitivity involves a physical overreaction to stimuli that is completely out of my control. For non-sufferers of M.E. it might be helpful to imagine the sensation of being extremely hung over. The smell of cooking that's so strong it wrenches up everything in your stomach. The first glimpse of stark daylight offending your eyes when you try to open them. The extreme irritability towards the ordinary sounds around you like the television or people trying to talk to you. Take those feelings and add to them an intense amount of physical pain when something just barely touches your skin, and you've got some kind of idea what hypersensitivity is like for people with M.E.

It's an incredibly irritating symptom of the condition for a number of reasons, the first being that it's totally invisible. Only you know you when it's starting to affect you: there's no magical red light bulb above your head to suddenly warn everyone around you to quiet down and keep their distance from you (though, frankly, I wish there was). The onset of being extremely sensitive to external stimuli creates a huge dilemma for me: if I tell people that I'm feeling hypersensitive, they tend to avoid me and/or walk on egg shells for the rest of the day. If I don't tell people how I'm feeling, they wonder why I'm losing my concentration and getting increasingly snappy and irritable with them. Either way it's going to upset my relationships with them for the current spell of symptoms.

From the outside view, there are only very subtle markers to let you know than an M.E. sufferer is going through a hypersensitive phase. I tend to narrow my eyes and my brow becomes quite heavily furrowed as the tension from the light around me increases. I also take my glasses on and off a lot, which I'm not usually prone to doing otherwise. I find that I sit in the most comfortable space that's farthest away from any televisions, windows or other sense-assaulting apparatus in the room, usually with one hand over my ear. If I put on a hoodie and pull the hood up to cover my brow and ears, then you know something really bad is going on. I also become extremely jumpy when people approach me or hand me things like mugs or plates because I know that the wrong pressure in the wrong place is going to cause pain and accidents that could be dangerous for everyone concerned.

Being involved in conversation is perhaps the biggest clue my nearest and dearest have for when I might need some quiet time in the corner. I tend not to involve myself in conversations with more than three participants in the first place because my brain fog (more on this lovely add-on condition later) doesn't allow me to stay focused on multiple threads of dialogue for very long, but hypersensitivity makes it hard to even talk to someone one on one. It's like my brain is trying to focus on the words that they're saying, but there are so many other sensations going on that it's hard to keep track. Here are a few examples of what could be happening at any given moment:

- The tone and volume of their words can be hurting my ears (even if they're speaking in a totally normal way).
- The speed at which they speak is causing me to miss words entirely which then stresses me out because I feel like I'm missing important things.
- Keeping focused on their face to show engagement with what they're saying is hard because of the light in the room

(sustaining focus under any kind of bright light, especially daylight, is extremely painful when I'm feeling hypersensitive).

- Even ordinary smells such as perfume or dust can be amplified, travelling down my nose and forming tastes on my tongue and at the back of my throat that make me feel sick.

- Any minor muscular or joint aches that I might have been having prior to hypersensitivity are now heightened to extremes and sending pain signals to my brain whilst I'm trying to concentrate.

- New pain sensations are being caused by ordinary harmless things like picking up a glass of water or sitting in the same position on a chair for too long (too long ranging anywhere from 30 minutes to 30 seconds depending on the severity of the sensitivity).

Is it any wonder that I sound 'off' and 'snappy' when I reply in these kinds of conversations? Out in the wider social world, invisible symptoms don't get much sympathy, but ultimately I've decided that it's probably better to forewarn people that I'm feeling hypersensitive, even if I do end up feeling like a lonely pariah because of it for the rest of the day. I'm fortunate that in my home environment I have people around me who will recognise the hoodie going up and endeavour to turn down the TV and block out as much light from the room as they can. It makes me feel incredibly guilty that they have to make these adjustments for me all the time, but it doesn't mean I'm not also terribly grateful for it. Turning the volume down tells me that they'd rather keep me in the room than banish me because I'm having symptoms and I believe that kind of consideration is something that every M.E. sufferer needs to have in their lives.

Temperature Control

or

'It's getting hot in here... but everyone else is wearing jumpers'

Let's begin this episode with a scene from my past. Picture it with me now. It is the Lake District in the middle of February. For those of you not familiar with British weather, this means it is bloody freezing and it's quite insane to be swanning about outdoors with frozen winds biting at you and ice, snow and frost scattered everywhere you look. The person with me is wearing a thermal t-shirt, a fleece and a jacket zipped up to his chin. He also sports a hat and a pair of thick gloves. We are not at any kind of altitude, merely standing beside a small pond on a wooden dock of sorts. I am posing for a photograph whilst we have some sunlight amid the clouds.

I'm wearing a t-shirt and thin jeans. No gloves, no hat, no scarf. Just me in my summer gear, surrounded by snow, the pond totally frozen over behind me. The person with me asks why I won't put my coat on. My answer?

"I'm really not cold."

This moment was pre-diagnosis and, at the time, I didn't even think of it as a symptom of M.E.; it seemed to me to just be a quirk of my personality that I was always the wrong temperature for my surroundings. I knew full well that I had pain and fatigue and other problems in my body, but I had never even heard of the word *homeostasis* at the time. Some years later, when I was in the process of being diagnosed, I came across that term on a website that stated that patients with M.E. had little or no control over the regulation of their body temperatures. I wondered in amazement as to why I hadn't considered that before.

Being unaware of my lack of temperature control had caused me several health problems that I wasn't even aware of. Because my feet were often extremely cold even when they shouldn't have been I hardly ever left them bare, wrapping them up in so many layers that I inadvertently reduced their oxygen supply. This left me open to the beginning stages of frostbite where my toes were numb for days on end. This also put my toenails into a sorry state, making them highly susceptible to infections and reducing healthy growth, a problem that has taken me over five years to rectify. I'm still not quite there now.

Awareness is often a huge problem for people with M.E. as our bodies don't tend to give us the correct signals about what's actually going on inside us. Not being able to tell if you're the right temperature leads to sunburn, sunstroke, chilblains, frostbite and various internal muscle aches from overexposure to the wrong atmosphere. It becomes necessary to rely on those around you to see what kind of clothes you should be wearing and what precautions you ought to take, even if you can't see the dangers for yourself.

This lack of homeostasis also presents a lovely array of social problems as well as its physical side effects. The inappropriate arrival of fevers, sweats and chills is always lurking around the corner in the rare occasions where I am out and about with the normal folk. There are few things more embarrassing than having everyone in a nice cool room stare at you because your face and hair are soaking wet and there are huge dark patches of sweat all over your clothes. It makes people shift their chairs away from you when they think you're not looking at them. But you are looking. You do notice. And it stings to know that people don't want to be near you for reasons they don't even understand.

The fevers that M.E. sufferers get aren't necessarily like the fevers you'd recognise in someone with the flu or any other condition (although they sometimes get those kinds of flare-ups too). Quite often the rest of my body temperature is so cold that the 'fever' in my head actually feels like it's a perfectly normal temperature, which makes you look like you're exaggerating when you say you're burning up. The thing that few non-sufferers can understand is how wrong your body's signals can be. It's possible to feel like every part of you is on fire in a wild raging fever, but have your skin be a completely normal temperature to touch.

Imagine walking down the street and seeing a mime doing the glass box routine. You smile for a moment at him and his look of total anguish, thinking he's very convincing. What if he actually *is* suffocating inside a glass box and you've just passed him by without helping him, simply because you can't see the box? A lack of homeostasis is an internal problem that messes with the messages your body's getting. It makes your body look like that glass box, so it seems, to the casual observer, that all your suffering is for nothing, or that everything is perfectly fine and you're just making things seem worse than they are.

It's been important for me to explain to those responsible for my care that I might not be aware of doing damage to myself in the wrong temperature situation. Having your mum remind you to put your coat on might seem a little backward for a woman of twenty-five, but believe me, it helps. It's not always a picnic for my friends when they come to visit in the middle of winter and find me sweating and refusing to put the heating on, but we manage somehow. The more we work together on finding the right conditions to keep me happy, the closer I get to feeling less guilty about my condition.

As with most things related to M.E., awareness is the word of the day when it comes to temperature control. If people know that this condition isn't just about being tired all the time, if they understand how it causes such extensive damage to the insides of your body, then perhaps they'll be a little less inclined to shuffle away when we're sweating it out and a little more inclined to open a window and help us regain our dignity.

Random Agony

or

'Why me God? Why me?'

M.E. is an unpredictable condition. That's one of the reasons why it makes it so hard for sufferers to sustain normal life-things like regular work and relationships with friends and partners. I regularly plan to do things and usually (if I've accounted for all the possibilities of what could go wrong) I can manage to do everything that I've planned. There is one symptom of my condition, however, that can prevent even the best laid plans from going ahead. I like to call it Random Agony.

Random Agony is my term for the sudden onset of pain and suffering that I get when there has been no identifiable cause for it. If I've done something stupidly daring like carrying a shopping bag or standing up for a while to help cook a meal, then I can understand where my pain has come from and remind myself not to be so foolish in future. Random Agony isn't like that. It simply shows up (usually first thing in the morning, but sometimes at other parts of the day) and manifests all over your body like you've been run over by a bus, leaving you wondering where the heck that bus came from and why you didn't see it hurtling towards you.

One of the biggest fears I have when I go to sleep is that I might not be able to walk when I wake up in the morning. Now that I have reduced my physical activity hours to their bare minimum, this terrifying state doesn't happen to me as often as it used to. When I was teaching or attending university for 7-9 hour days, I could pretty much predict that I wouldn't have any strength in my legs the next day to get about on my own, so it was a less of a shock to wake up feeling that way. Random Agony brings back the feelings I had in those healthier days and it is my number one fear when I lie in the darkness trying to sleep.

Imagine this with me for a moment.

You are lying in your bed, slowly coming back to consciousness in the morning light after a perfectly ordinary yesterday and a fairly restful night's sleep. You shuffle about, attempting to lift your head off the pillow to see what time it is. A shocking pain like the rumble of a horrific hangover wracks the back of your skull. You groan and sink back into the pillow, fearful of the moment when you have to lift your head totally and feel the full effect of the strain. Instead, you try to stretch your legs out so you can get up gradually. What's this? It seems someone has tied lead weights to your ankles, knees and hips. Your legs want to move, but you feel as though you're dragging dead weight around every time you shift them. Your torso and arms feel much the same and the effort from trying to move them makes it feel like someone has snuck in and surgically removed one of your lungs in the night. You are exhausted after the smallest motion. Your head is so sore it threatens to burst like a rotten melon if you lift it again. You are immobile and trapped in a world of pain. Worse still, you are so breathless you can't even shout for someone to help you.

Welcome to Random Agony.

It's no wonder we M.E. sufferers get a bit depressed sometimes. I consider myself fortunate now that my life is arranged in such a way that these horrific episodes are fewer and further between, but living with the possibility of being struck down in that way is no picnic either. Being in the grip of such a terrible sensation makes you want to cry and scream at God or Fate (or your all powerful deity of choice) and ask them why they chose to you to be the bearer of such an incredible burden. I'm still waiting on an answer to that one; if I get one, I'll let you know.

Ultimately, calling out to the almighty isn't the solution. Random Agony in my life is a case of 'prevention is better than cure'. I have spent years arranging my life in the right way so that I don't deliberately do things to encourage it, which reduces the problem considerably but doesn't eradicate it. I know I will still be struck down if my body feels like shutting off for a day or two (sometimes longer), and I will still cry and scream about it when it first hits me like I always do. But, when I'm over that, I try to keep things in perspective.

M.E. is an ever-changing condition. And that means things don't tend to last very long when they attack you. Fatigue and pain are a permanent given, but everything else has a shelf life on it. Whatever this random happening of pain is, it will not last. It may be frustrating and it may be upsetting, but it will come to an end. Whatever good things this attack has prevented me from doing, I can catch up on them and make up for lost time when it has passed. I have to repeat that last one to myself a few times before it sinks in.

For me, it's not even the pain or the unexpected nature of the illness that gets to me; it's the way that it interrupts my plans. I am a person who likes to feel purposeful, to know when I lie down to sleep at night that I have done something each day to contribute to making my life or the life of someone I know a little better. Spending all day swaddled in blankets crying in agony doesn't rate high on the purposeful scale; if anything I always feel worse for being a burden to those around me. The important thing that I try to hang onto is that it isn't my fault that I feel this way. Trying to remain functional when my body is under attack would only lead me to much more serious health problems if I were to push myself too far.

Good things come to those who wait. Patience is a virtue. Those old, overused sayings are old and overused for a reason. They're true. And it doesn't hurt to repeat them to yourself once in a while when Random Agony gets you down.

Balance

or

'Every step is a tightrope walk'

Let's be clear about this section before I start it: this isn't a chapter about getting your life in balance or something on those lines. This is about falling over a lot, something many people with M.E. struggle with but aren't that inclined to admit to. It's one of the most invisible of all the symptoms that we have to deal with, until you suddenly find yourself on the floor with everybody staring at you. For some people it only affects them in little ways, for others it can be a far more dangerous thing.

I tend to do things differently when I'm left in the house on my own. When my fabulous support system of mum and best friend are called away by their other life duties, my attitude towards my existence changes a little. When they're not here to do things for me and tell me to sit still whilst they fetch and carry, I get a little too ambitious for my own good. I lift things I shouldn't lift, I climb and reach for stuff that I ought to wait until later for and, perhaps most importantly for this chapter, I move around a lot faster.

I'm usually working when I have the house to

myself. Mum leaves me snacks in easy reach and I sit with my computer and write, getting up to stretch, breathe and visit the bathroom or the kettle depending on which biological urge is stronger at the time. I get very engrossed in my work and my mind races with more ideas than I actually have time to write down, so when I get up to do things I am always in a hurry to get back to the keyboard and continue my frantic scribblings before the ideas fade away. As such, I rush along the corridors of our flat.

Rushing is not a practice that goes hand in hand with having M.E. since poor circulation and constant headaches make it hard for us to retain our physical balance at the best of times. When I rush, my brain loses control of what my feet are doing and can't relay information fast enough between my eyes and my legs. So I fall over a lot. Most of the time the bruises are in places that my family can't see them, so I don't need to mention the falls unless they've stopped me walking or injured me in a more severe way, like the time I tripped on a coffee table and slashed my leg open a little.

I frequently misjudge doorframes and furniture, even when I'm not at liberty to rush about pretending to be a healthy, busy person. Walking into things doesn't make the best impression in social situations either, which makes me sincerely glad that I'm no longer in the world of education, classrooms and their associated social hierarchies. People have a gut reaction to find physical accidents funny; that's the whole basis of the genre of slapstick comedy. It's just not as funny when it's happening to *you* personally.

It also breeds a terrible kind of nervousness about putting one foot in front of the other. I don't like to walk too close to pavement edges, for example, and I find I'm a lot more afraid to cross the road than anyone else I know. Perhaps that's because they're only afraid of wayward traffic, whereas I have to be concerned about my own body letting me down and making me collapse in the road in front of some poor unsuspecting driver. It's not an unfounded fear: I have been clipped a few times when my legs have just decided to make the wrong motion when I'm part-way across a junction.

You're starting to see why I stay indoors a lot, aren't you?

Here's a simple sum. Bad Nerves + Bad Balance = Clumsiness.

Here's an even simpler sum. Clumsiness = Personal Danger.

That last one has some worrying complications. Clumsiness doesn't just mean putting myself in physical danger if I drop or break something because of my condition. It also makes me feel stupid and useless. Maybe some people don't care if they drop a glass and it shatters, but I really, really care when it happens to me. It makes me feel like I can't trust myself and like others can't trust me. I still prefer to drink cold drinks from my Pyrex Pokémon mug that I was given when I was about twelve. If I didn't, then a set of six new table glasses would rapidly become a set of five, four, three (and so on) before my very eyes. It's patronising to be the one holding the sippy cup like a toddler, but it's necessary when your nerves are acting up.

A lot of people are able to relate to M.E. sufferers in terms of the physical pain that they go through and the crippling fatigue they feel, but not a lot of people stop to think about the personal dignity of someone with a debilitating condition. For me, balance is all about dignity, it's about becoming aware of the times when you're going to trip up and make an ass of yourself so that you can avoid and prevent them as often as possible. But it's also about letting the people you trust in on your secrets: allowing yourself the humility to admit to them that you might need help in a particular task in case you hurt yourself doing it.

There's nothing undignified about asking for help when you really need it.

The final step in that journey, one that I'm aware of but have not yet mastered, is admitting that you still need help even when you're alone. You need to help yourself stay well by admitting that there are some things you need to watch out for. Patience and self-restraint are qualities that I'm improving on slowly as I get older, because learning not to be in a hurry all the time is the obvious solution to not being covered in bruises every day. More than that though, taking time out to consider my lot in life and give help to myself is the obvious solution to learning to cope with my condition as a whole.

Anxiety

or

'Not letting the frogs out of the box'

I am a terribly anxious person. Even before I had M.E., I was an extremely nervous child who constantly worried about eventualities that other people couldn't even see. If I saw kids playing a ball game in the school playground, I would walk with my tongue stuck to the roof of my mouth and my teeth gritted together. Why? Because if I *happened* to have my tongue between my teeth and their ball *happened* to hit me in the jaw, I'd bite the end of my tongue off, of course. These are the kinds of things I used to worry about constantly and unfortunately the tongue-habit has stayed with me now, even though I know that particular nightmare isn't likely to come true.

M.E. does some serious messing with a person's nerves. The nervous system is one of the major systems that the condition affects, causing trouble in terms of increased pain signals, adrenaline rushes, twitches and sleep disturbances. In short, it sends your nerves into overdrive. People who are subject to anxiety and stress in their lives fall into the category of 'people who are likely to develop M.E.', so it's a nasty blow for someone who already has anxiety problems to suddenly have their nerves frazzled by an illness on top of that. It's little wonder I was misdiagnosed with depression and anxiety for such a long time before we worked out what was really going on.

One thing that I have come to understand about anxiety is that it is a process which starts in the brain. Having a good relationship with your brain and how it works is a good first step to learning to control anxiety. For a start, I have made a big focus in my life on reducing my adrenaline levels. Adrenaline is a chemical reaction set off by exposing your body to undue stress and/or exertion and it's a big problem for M.E. sufferers. For me, opening a milk bottle counts as exertion, so it does prove difficult to keep your body chemistry in check when day to day activities can let absurd amounts of adrenaline build up in your system. It's a question of being self-aware and remembering to slow down so that you don't make a bad situation any worse for yourself.

It's not just for my mental clarity that I do this either. In recent years I have had serious problems with heart palpitations, which I now understand were caused by my own overexertion and the release of copious amounts of adrenaline that my heart couldn't cope with. I could be sitting completely still watching television (or even lying down in bed trying to sleep) and suddenly I'd have a surge in my chest as though I'd just gotten off a rollercoaster. The first time it happened, I genuinely thought I was going to die. I used to get up in the night and get into bed with my mother so that I could calm down enough to sleep (not a dignified thing to admit, since I was nineteen at the time). It was painful and frightening for me and my family to have to deal with and, at the time, I had no idea that M.E. was to blame for it.

Anxiety makes a sick body even sicker. It eats up energy that I could be using to do other more constructive things. It upsets my stomach so that I can't keep food down when I really need to eat to sustain myself. It hurts my heart and lungs, putting them under terrible strain that, if left uncontrolled, will lead me to serious trouble in later years. So anxiety is not something I want in my life: it has to go.

But that's easier said than done. A lot of people suffer from anxiety whether they have other medical conditions or not. Some would see it as a sudden, overwhelming sensation that comes over them like a puppet master pulling their strings as they lose all control of their reactions. I see it as an ice cold pair of hands that picks me up by the heart and shakes the heck out of me, making me feel like they're never going to let go. The important thing I have to tell myself is that the puppet strings *can* be cut and I *can* wriggle out of the cold hands' grip. I just have to remember the right method to achieve success.

Stress and strain are part of life: no matter how many things you arrange in order to stop that adrenaline from racing into your system, it's still going to leak through sometimes. My belief is to accept that reality and put steps in motion to deal with it when it happens. Remove yourself to a calm, comfortable place. Breathe deeply. Read a good book. Take a remedy you trust or have a hot cup of tea. When anxiety strikes, I try lots of different things to battle it until I find one that works, because sitting in the middle of a panic attack and worrying about it only prolongs the pain. At least by trying activities (even if they don't work), I feel as though I'm doing something about the anxiety and that I'm asserting some kind of control.

I suppose it's kind of like having faith in yourself. Anxiety, for me, is the fear of a lack of control over a situation (or the prospect of a stressful event). So by taking control of how I feel and trying to fix it, I'm reaffirming the belief in myself that I don't have to let anxiety be my master. Over time this faith has helped me to reduce my palpitations from three times daily to once monthly and improved my general mental health as well as my sleep and gastric/digestive problems. I'm not saying that it's been easy. It has taken a long time and I've had plenty of failed attempts at taking control along the way.

And I'm not saying that I'm by any means over my anxious thoughts. I'll still find my tongue stuck to the roof of my mouth if I pass too close to some kids playing football on the street, because I can't help the presence of that sudden, anxious idea. The difference now is that the anxious thought doesn't get the chance to translate into a reaction that could hurt my body, and the rare ones that do slip through the net will meet a whole arsenal of methods I have for eradicating them on the other side.

Depression

or

'Of course I feel sad - I'm ill!'

Depression has become a bit of a throwaway word in our society right now. The phrase 'I'm depressed' quite often replaces 'I'm sad' for such ordinary everyday situations as not getting a pair of jeans in your size or choosing a bad meal in a restaurant. There is a big difference between *feeling* depressed and *having* what is known as clinical depression. Clinical depression is a serious chemical defect in the brain that makes you feel as though you will never have the capacity to be happy again. In the case of people with long-term illnesses, both types of depression are likely to rear their ugly heads as time goes by.

There have been a lot of campaigns lately in the UK to make people less afraid of admitting that they have (or have had) mental illness and, in turn, to show the general public that 'ordinary' people can be sufferers of mental illness too. The message is supposed to be about not shunning people for conditions they can't help having, which I personally think is a great idea, but there's a lot of information about illnesses like depression which doesn't make it into the TV advert or the nice, glossy brochure.

One such fact is that clinical depression is the number one initial misdiagnosis given to people with M.E.

I was misdiagnosed with clinical depression when I was sixteen years old. Because my parents had recently broken up, the group of therapists I was sent to see made a unanimous decision that my tiredness, pain and extremely bitter attitude were a product of depression. They prescribed me some tablets and terminated my counselling sessions, effectively dusting their hands off and saying 'Well, that's her sorted out'. I had no better information to go on at the time, not even realising that conditions like M.E. existed, so I went along with their diagnosis and took the tablets regardless of whether I was feeling good or bad that day.

What I discovered is this: clinical depression brings with it a physical incapability to lift yourself out of a bad mood. When I was sixteen and apparently 'depressed', skipping school and buying a custard slice from the bakery on my way home made me feel on top of the world. Staying at home to watch TV, surf the internet and get a good afternoon's sleep (because I rarely slept at night in those days) solved virtually all my problems, for a time at least. The more I took my antidepressants, the more drowsy I became. I started to be too drowsy to enjoy the things I'd once enjoyed, spending entire days asleep in bed. I dropped out of sixth-form college in that same period because my mind was too addled to take anything in.

The mind is a powerful thing. I'm not going to sit here and blame the medication for making me feel as though I had depression, because I think the process of giving up on your vitality is far more complex than that. But being told that you have a condition *does* change the way you feel about yourself. I think being told I had depression was my first step on the road to actually getting it. This difficult period of my life lasted two years before I came off all anti-depressant tablets and realised that there was a lot more to my physical problem than the doctors initially told me.

One of the biggest problems with having clinical depression on your medical record is that doctors, at least most of the ones I've known, tend to hone in on it and want to blame every new symptom you get on it. I have completed more anxiety and depression surveys upon meeting new doctors than I care to remember, and I have to be very careful about how I answer them in order to get the professionals to focus on my M.E. rather than the black mark of depression in my past. If your doctors feel that you might have depression, I'd strongly recommend taking a good long look at yourself before you let them throw pills at you for it. The stigma afterwards is far more prominent than the TV adverts lead you to believe.

Feeling depressed, on the other hand, is something I know every M.E. sufferer will relate to. Frankly it astounds me when people are surprised that we sufferers have teary, moody days. We are completely exhausted, even with hours and hours of sleep at night. We are constantly in a state of physical strain just trying to lead a normal life. We have to consider precautions and assess our risk of suffering in all the everyday activities that other people take for granted. It's a hard way to live, and we have no choice about it. *Of course* we're going to feel sad more than once in a while!

The biggest concern my family and friends have for me is that this condition might force me to 'slip back' into the state of clinical depression every time I face a new period of deterioration. If I have a teary day, there always comes a moment when someone close to me will ask me if I feel that depression is around the corner. It's wonderful that they care enough to ask, but really I get sick of having to say 'No, I'm not depressed' every time I feel that I need a good cry. Crying all the time because of a chronic illness does not mean that you have depression. Self-awareness is the key to knowing when the real alarm bells might start to ring.

I have projects going. I may be unemployed in a physical, going-out-to-work sense, but I am a writer and a distance-learning student with goals and deadlines for things that have to be done. When I was truly depressed, I cancelled every goal from my life, every single thing that indicated that I might be looking towards the future, because I was too consumed by the intense sadness of the immediate moment to look beyond it. Sure, there are times when I get stressed and want to throw in the towel nowadays, but everybody has times like that when the world gets on top of them. The reason I know I'm not medically depressed is because I overcome those moments and carry on achieving the goals I've set to improve my health and my life.

Sadness is a natural part of being constantly ill, but if you can still see the light at the end of the tunnel, then depression doesn't have to be an inevitable thing.

Emotional Pain

or

'Being your own worst enemy'

In the previous section, a lesson was learned that 'clinical depression' and 'feeling depressed' are not the same thing, but depression, low moods and anxiety are not the only horrible emotions that can encroach on the life of an M.E. sufferer. For me there are plenty of other bugbears that cloud my mind and cause me aggravation on a daily basis such as mood swings (both high and low), irritation, tearfulness and pure, undiluted rage.

I can imagine that a healthy person reading this might say 'So what?' to the above. These are all normal emotions that most people go through in their daily lives: they get teary over a sad movie, they scream at the computer because it's crashed in the middle of something important, or their mood rises and falls with the company they keep and the situation they're in. It's perfectly normal to go through a wide range of emotions in your daily life. But here's a thought:

What if your emotions were directly related to your physical health?

When you have M.E., you spend a lot of time thinking about energy. I have thoughts like: 'When I get up for the toilet, I'll fetch a drink as well so I don't need to get up twice'. Everything you do is about physical conservation. We directly relate movement to energy all the time. Something I realised all too late is this:

Emotions cost energy too.

The extreme highs and lows of emotional states are huge energy-suckers. You could lie in bed resting all day long, but if you're lying there feeling extremely distressed and upset, your physical condition will not improve. You could also sit still at a dinner table for a long time in relative comfort, but if you're engaged in constant conversation with your friends and roaring with fits of hysterical laughter, later on you're going to find that you feel very ill from a strain you didn't even know was happening.

I spend about 95% of my time sitting around in my flat, but I still find that I have dramatic highs and lows in both mood and energy, even though I'm not going out and doing things. This is because even when my body is resting, my mind is still active, sometimes even more so because my physical state is so inert. Personally, I know that I have a very over-active mind with massive tendencies towards stress and worry. That is a separate issue to my M.E. that I am still working on, and one that drains my emotions constantly. But there are other causes of emotional energy-drain that I know fellow sufferers have described too.

Distress. Resentment. Build-up of sad feelings over time. Worthlessness. Pretending to be fine. Denial. Guilt. Hysteria-like merriment caused by adrenaline.

Having an illness that affects everything you do is not an easy thing to live with. You are definitely going to struggle emotionally. It's normal to feel all of the frustrations listed above and so many more. The difficult part is not letting those feelings affect you so deeply that your health suffers because of it. Having family and friends in the equation makes things difficult too: if you're suffering, they worry; if you're hiding the fact that you're suffering, you don't get the support that you need. And they still worry, even if you think you're looking and acting fine. They will always worry once you have this condition and you will always feel guilty about that, because emotions are natural things that come to you whether you want them to or not.

There is no amazing secret trick to mastering the way you feel about your condition. Acceptance of myself was a huge breakthrough for me. Once I fully allowed myself to be seen as a disabled person, I found that I was less afraid to ask for and accept help, as well as more willing to fight for my rights and those of others that I know. Some people find it extremely helpful to record their thoughts, both positive and negative, in a diary and then try to redirect them on the page into something more balanced. I suppose, in a way, that's what I'm doing as I write this book.

Whatever you do to get in charge of your feelings, it has to be proactive.

Emotions do pass in time, but all the time while you're waiting for that horrible, heavy sadness to pass by, it's eating away at valuable energy that you could have used to do other more enjoyable things. If you can nip a particular emotion in the bud by stopping what you're doing or leaving a certain situation, then you have every right to do so. In the middle of a lively conversation or an over-stimulating TV show with my family and friends, I often have to get up and say 'Sorry, I've got to go to my room for five minutes'. Once I'm on my own, I'll try a few different things to make that feeling pass, whether they are relaxation techniques, like breathing, or distraction techniques, like reading a few pages of a good book until the emotion goes away.

Being proactive about the condition helps more than I first realised. Yes, I'm in a bad situation, but at least I'm doing something about it. However small my effort, it's a step in the right direction.

For my family and friends, the most important thing they can do is just allow me to have my moment. They don't understand half of what I'm feeling; it's impossible for them to process all of the complex emotions that pass through my head every day that I live with pain and total exhaustion. The situation is never truly imaginable if you don't have M.E., but acceptance is a much easier feat to achieve regardless of how much you understand. A combination of personal proactivity and sympathetic support can go a long way to not letting your emotions get the better of you.

Self Esteem

or

'I'm here, I'm crippled, get used to it'

Having any kind of disability doesn't exactly make you feel like the coolest kid on the block but M.E., as we have discovered, has a fabulous selection of embarrassing add-on symptoms to choose from that breed chaos and humiliation wherever you go. It's embarrassing for a lot of healthy people to have to adjust to 'special considerations' being made for them when they suddenly become ill. If you break your arm, for example, and your partner has to cut up your food because you can't hold your knife, you might feel a little bit less competent as a human being for a while. If you have to wear a very visible bandage, splint or cast, you might be upset that people keep asking you all the time if you're okay.

You might just want to feel like everyone else, even though your life's a little different to theirs.

This book talks a lot about raising awareness as to what M.E. is really like for its sufferers, but I'm not trying to arrange a nationwide Sympathy Parade. If you read it all and you have some understanding of the terrible difficulties that we sufferers have to go through every day, then that's wonderful, but it doesn't mean you have to put us on a pedestal because of it. Most M.E. sufferers that I know just want to get on with their lives in the best way that they can. They don't need coddling or wrapping up in bubble wrap. They just want you to give them a break now and then, and be understanding when things go wrong, because for us, they often do.

Self-esteem can mean many things. It can mean finding a purposeful place in the world of work by being part of a team or doing a good job. It can mean feeling good about the way that you physically look. It can mean being a good relative or friend and being there for the people that matter to you. It can mean feeling good about the person you are inside and how you represent that to the world. The condition causes M.E. sufferers to have problems in all of these areas. These are some of mine by example:

My physical state is such a mess that I can't work in a real-world environment, so I have no regular social team to be part of. I do contact my colleagues and peers in the writing world via social networks, but then I also have to see all the amazing things they go out and achieve every day, so my self-esteem is damaged by believing that their quality of life is far better than mine. I feel like I'm missing out on my life.

My physical appearance is marred by unsightly additions that my condition has caused. I have dark circles around my eyes from fatigue. I am about three stone overweight for my height. I have horrible protruding veins on the upper part of my legs from the physical strain of walking when my muscles aren't up to scratch. Thanks to immune systems problems caused by fatigue, I have spots that turn septic and take weeks to heal, often turning into boils that leave me with blemishes and scars that then take years to fade away. My self-esteem is damaged because I know this illness is doing permanent damage to my looks that I can't reverse. I feel ugly and worthless.

When my friends and family are in need, I am not the person they call for help. They know that they can't rely on me to always be there, even though I sorely want to assist them. Sometimes they can't even trust my physical skills to withstand the task they need to accomplish. Lines like 'You don't actually have to help me do this, just sit there and keep me company' spring to mind. My self-esteem is damaged because I can't repay the constant kindnesses and attention that they give me. I feel like a bad friend.

My personality is variable because of my moods. I get snappy and irritable and I lash out at people for no reason except that my pain is so extreme that it needs an outlet. I am frustrated with myself for the countless cognitive problems that are caused by my fatigue and I vent those frustrations on people who are only trying to help me overcome them. I can be aggressive and hysterically upset, watching my family and friends stare at me helplessly because I can't keep a lid on how I feel. My self-esteem is damaged because I can't help hurting them. They deserve better than me. I feel like a bad person, inside and out.

I'm sure there are plenty of other ways that self-esteem issues can destroy a person's hope and zest for life, but I think I've listed quite enough of my surface emotions here without digging for more. These are thoughts that I have every single day when my condition gets in the way of my life and brings them all to mind.

That doesn't mean they have to become who I am.

But I can't be like everyone else either. I am different, no matter how much I wish I wasn't. M.E. has claimed me and branded me with its mark. Lives being lived all around me suggest all the 'normal' things I should be doing, but I can't do them. If you boil it down cynically, then people come in three categories: ignorant, judgemental, or overly-sympathetic. I am stuck in a world that isn't designed for my way of living, struggling not to fall into a black hole of inadequacy because of everything I see around me.

So how do I carry on with all that is weighing down on me?

I stop comparing myself to that world.

My life is my own world to create. I can set the standard by which I feel purposeful in my working life. I can show off my best skills and my achievements in writing to my peers and even have them be envious of all the time I have at home to work and write and promote. I can decide the benchmark for my own level of personal beauty by buying clothes that flatter my overweight shape and working to disguise those parts of me that are damaged by my illness. I can prepare to help my nearest and dearest by resting up ready to assist them and by pacing myself every day so that if they need to call on me, I'm there.

Perhaps most importantly, I can decide the things which make me a good person in the eyes of those around me. I can celebrate the fact that I bothered to get out of bed this morning despite the tear-inducing agony of dragging myself upright. I can celebrate the fact that I managed to get some writing done despite my headache and the pains in my wrists from typing. I can celebrate the fact that I push through boundaries every single day of my life to go on living, achieving and fighting to find a purposeful place in society despite my condition.

Self-esteem isn't about matching up to what other people have; it's about appreciating what *you* have and *celebrating* those things every day. There are plenty of things to feel proud of if you take the time to refocus your energy on looking for them, instead of letting yourself drown in a pretend world of what might have been.

Headaches

or

'There's definitely something wrong with my brain'

Last night I had a horrible, life-halting headache. After a relatively busy day in which I used my brain quite a lot, it suddenly decided to go into a pain-riddled overdrive and ruin what should have been a relaxing night with my family. M.E. tends to put its own special stamp on every area of illness that it touches, and the specifics of the M.E. headache are no exception to that rule. From my perspective, I see the M.E. headache as a blend of tiredness, physical pain, emotional stress, anxiety and hypersensitivity that leaves my head aching with an overload of thoughts that I can't quieten down.

Having multiple causes for a headache means that there's no single, perfect solution to getting rid of it once it's taken hold of you. You can sleep for tiredness, but not if you're also having anxiety and hypersensitivity. You can take painkillers for physical pain, but that won't alleviate emotional stress. You can breathe deep and try relaxation methods for the anxiety, but they won't necessary relieve the actual thumping of the strained capillaries in your skull. Frustration sets in, adding anger to the mix. Family and friends try to help, but there's little they can do, making you feel even more upset that you've got them worrying and fretting as well.

My solution last night? Lie around in agony until it goes away. For a period of about two hours, there was literally nothing more I could try and do to take away that kind of overload pain; I simply had to wait until it had faded enough to do something to take my mind off the rest of the ache. The sad truth about M.E. treatment is that sometimes, there is no solution to the problem. The only solace you have is knowing that the condition is an ever-changing one, and that the worst pains in the mix don't last forever.

The real solution is a tried and tested adage: Prevention is better than cure.

Sometimes you can't help having an overload kind of day, because life throws things at you that you need to sort out, and it has a nasty habit of piling them all onto the same day too. Yesterday, to be honest with you, I could easily have prevented that horrifying headache, but I took a chance that I wouldn't get one and it backfired with gusto. I shouldn't have taken so much on in one day. I should have planned appropriate rest in between activities. I should have used my medication to ward off the early physical signs of decline before that headache ever got started.

With a condition like this, you learn how to cope as

you go along. In conversations with people who have had M.E. for as long as me, I find that we tend to be able to categorise our different kinds of headaches based on their cause. There's the stress-headache which usually features pain in the temples and forehead, the tiredness-headache which begins with a burning sensation behind the eyes, the physical-exertion-headache which pounds out your pulse in the space where your neck meets your skull: the list really is endless once you get going. To the casual observer, it probably seems like a very depressing thing to do, but it's actually a vital part of getting to understand the signals that your body is trying to give you.

This is because sometimes we get headaches that are nothing to do with M.E. as well, and we'd be in big trouble if we couldn't tell the difference. Headaches are the body's way of saying that something is wrong: they can be precursors of illnesses, infections and/or exposure to unsafe stimuli like fumes, noise and even bad food. Having a chronic illness sometimes means that you have the tendency to lump all your symptoms together and, for many years, I ignored the possibility that there were other, easily-treatable, things adding to my usual pain. Had I been able to recognise and treat those things separately, I would have saved myself a lot of hassle.

Headaches aren't the only thing that this theory applies to; there are plenty of other kinds of pain and discomfort that an M.E. sufferer needs to be aware of and be able to identify as 'not what I usually deal with'. If you can analyse your body and break down what you normally feel and how you normally treat it, then you can start to pick out those extra things that don't fit the pattern and find new ways of dealing with them. Some people like to keep thought records to jot this stuff down. For me, it's just about taking a few minutes out of my day to ask myself 'How am I feeling? Is there anything extra going on that I need to deal with?'

When I forget to do that incredibly simple thing, I end up in agony like I did last night, as all the different forms of headache creep up on me to produce the monster version that takes over your life for hours on end. This morning, I can try to let those wasted hours slide and be content at least that I eventually managed to settle down for some sleep. I know for certain now that that kind of headache won't hit me again for a week at least. That's not because I have some magical foreknowledge of my body, but because the experience was so horrible that *I won't let it* hit me again. Whilst the memory of those agonising hours is fresh, I will be on the lookout for ways to prevent it from reoccurring. The next time it happens will be a day when I'm too busy to do that, or too consumed by a project to remember the price I'm going to pay for not taking a break.

Every day with this unpredictable illness is a learning experience and a lesson in life management that will hopefully lead me to make better choices in the future. That is, of course, so long as I'm willing to pay attention to what my body's trying to tell me.

Brain Fog

or

'I'm clever really, honest I am.'

I am a teacher, or at least I still think like one, even if my condition has put a stop to any actual teaching for the time being. As a teacher of the English Language, I always prided myself on eloquence when speaking: the accuracy of my language and the way I got my point across had me branded as a 'natural teacher' before I'd even left university. As a writer too, there is a certain expectation when people speak to me that I will have a special 'way with words' based on the craftsmanship I put into my novels.

Well, I have a confession to make:

I have Brain Fog.

Brain Fog is a popular term among M.E. sufferers for the various cognitive difficulties that we get. These can include (but are not limited to) problems in sustaining concentration, lapses in memory, speech impediments and symptoms akin to dyslexia and dyscalculia. A lot of people are surprised to find that M.E. patients have cognitive difficulties but, if you think about it, being exhausted and in pain all the time is bound to affect your ability to process things. If you hadn't slept all night and had a slamming headache, would you be 100% happy and able to have a spritely conversation at the breakfast table the next morning? I think not.

Brain Fog is something that first affected me when I was at high school, before I ever knew I even had a medical condition. To contextualise this, I'd like you to know that I was an outstanding academic student and frequently given prizes for being the best in various subjects all throughout my schooldays. So when, at about age 15, my mind suddenly went blank and I had no idea what I'd just listened to for an entire hour in my maths class, I was a little more than disturbed by my brain switching itself off without my permission.

I started falling asleep in class, something I was mortified by and admittedly frightened of. I couldn't remember questions that we'd been set five minutes ago, and having to ask my neighbouring students what we were supposed to be doing was highly embarrassing for the kid who was always top of the class. I wasn't popular to begin with, but now I was even stranger than before. I was able to study hard (at home and independently) for my exams and do well in them, but my in-class grades and behaviour were a mess. Lucky for me (or not, depending on how I look at it now) The misdiagnosis of clinical depression happened at same time, so I wasn't heavily punished for these issues by my educators.

Eventually I dropped out of education for eighteen months and, when I returned to do my A-Levels and a university degree, I found that I could study most of the work in peace at home and then, if I tuned out in class, it wouldn't be too much of an issue. It didn't build good relationships with my new educators, but it helped me get by and succeed in a way that was suitable for me. If I'd had my diagnosis sooner, it might have helped them to understand my needs better, but I made it eventually all the same.

Brain Fog is most prevalent in large, busy gatherings, so classrooms are an ideal spot for the M.E. mind to go blank. In my teaching years I discovered that I was best suited to small class and one-to-one teaching because it meant I was less likely to lose the thread of what I was trying to say and therefore (hopefully) not confuse my students either. Situations that were likely to send my stress levels through the roof encouraged serious problems with my ability to speak; I still can't hold telephone conversations now because my hearing isn't brilliant and the stress of listening hard makes me fearful that I'm going to get all my words wrong when it's my turn to reply.

There are still two things about Brain Fog that irritate me. The first is that it has made me a dyslexic typist. Every other word I type comes out wrong, which is a slight problem when your primary profession involves writing thousands of words every month. When I say wrong, I don't just mean two letters swapped over either. I mean letters that don't even belong in the word and extra words that have banana entered my mind and slipped into the sentence without me realising it (see what I did there). I joke now, but really it's no laughing matter. When I'm up against a deadline and I have to retype every single sentence and proofread until my eyes bleed, it's a very sad and frustrating thing. The laptop gets a lot of abuse from me for this very reason.

I have started to notice it happening in my handwritten notes too, something that I've never encountered before, but that's another issue for another time I think (see the section on dealing with deterioration later on).

The second thing that really winds me up is when I say the wrong thing in the middle of a sentence. It's just so embarrassing. People who don't know that I have this condition (and even the less-informed ones that do) look at me like I've got three heads if I mistakenly say 'can' instead of 'can't' or 'house the roundeds' instead of 'round the houses'. It just doesn't fit when I'm actually talking about quite complex and important things. I also have a tendency to trail off in the middle of a sentence because I've simply lost the end of what I intended to say, which makes me feel as though a sinkhole needs to develop under my feet and suck me away with it as soon as possible. It makes me feel stupid.

But I'm not stupid.

Nobody with Brain Fog is actually stupid or limited in any way. Just because we don't think in the same way as everyone else, it doesn't mean we can't think just as well or be just as creative, logical or practical. We have to find a new way to do the things that non-sufferers take for granted, like listening, speaking, taking phone calls and addressing friends. I embrace my Brain Fog proudly as I would an annoying little brother, for without it and the challenges it's brought me, I wouldn't know how smart I truly am for overcoming it.

Sleep

or

'How I learned to nod off'

In a condition where fatigue is the primary symptom that causes most of your other problems, you may think that M.E. patients generally don't sleep very well. I sleep about eight hours a night like any other person. I am very restless and I have pains and discomforts which sometimes wake me up, but generally I'd say my sleep is about as good as it's going to get. But every morning I wake up as though I've only had twenty minutes good sleep all night. This has nothing to do with the quality of my actual sleep; this is because one of the principal diagnosing factors of M.E. is 'fatigue that does not improve with rest'.

I have been through a lot of different stages of coping with sleep problems in my life and I feel that it's this bizarre journey of changing habits that finally led me to become an M.E. sufferer who can proudly say that she rarely ever has trouble with sleep any more. It is my hope that outlining some of these various patterns of sleep in my life will enable others to spot bad habits in themselves or the people that they are reading this book for. If they're lucky, then maybe they can skip a few stages and get to the healthy sleep part much faster than I did.

Let's take the clock back to stage one, when I was aged 13 to 16. This was the daytime sleep phase, in which I came home from school at four o'clock and went straight to bed, too tired to even change out of my school uniform before I fell asleep. This was the stage where I dozed off in class with alarming regularity. This was the stage where I was so tired that I came home early from school (without permission) in order to catch up on my sleep. At this time I was hardly sleeping at night, though I lay there in my bed most nights and tried to sleep all the same. I came to a point in this stage where I just started staying up half the night anyway because I knew I wasn't going to get to sleep: a move which only increased the vicious cycle and made my life even harder to lead.

I have often been heard to say that I sleep better in the day than I do at night. When I have monitored my sleep by way of an electronic tracker, my body is much more still and restful between the hours of sunrise and waking than it is when I first settle in the dark phase of the night. This is no excuse for staying up all night and sleeping my day away because, even if it's true, I know now that I'm wasting the time when I should be awake and involved with the world. If I could go back to that earlier me, she and I would find a way to calm her mind at night so that things could be a bit more balanced for her.

Stage two of my sleep journey was drug-induced. I was prescribed anti-depressants, which made me incredibly drowsy, and I later went on to use other tranquilisers for my anxiety problems which also made me extremely heavy-headed. This stage lasted from the ages of 17 to roughly 21. You might think that being given drowsy drugs at night meant that I then suddenly made a switch from sleeping all day to sleeping all night, leaving my days free to go back to normal and functional. Instead, I found that I was sleeping both all night *and* all day. Every chance I had to put my head down and nap, I took it.

This was most noticeable when I was at college. I sometimes had lessons from 9:30 a.m. to 11 a.m., then my next lesson wouldn't be until 2:30 p.m., so I was inclined to get the bus home, sleep two hours, then get the bus back rather than stay on campus with my friends. This was a completely regular and normal life for me at the time, especially being undiagnosed and avoiding doctors. Later in this same period, I frequently missed my stop getting to university because I didn't wake up until the bus had turned the corner a long way down the road from the campus buildings. I tried to be late with a casual sort of carelessness rather than admit that I was too heavily sedated to know where I was on my bus route.

I got sick of keeping up this façade, especially as my workload and pressures at university increased. I needed more clear-mind time than I had because I was always half-asleep, so I ceased taking any and all medication that had the potential to make me drowsy. This was stage three: the insomnia stage, brought about by anxiety, which lasted through ages 22 to 24. In this stage a lot of the nerve problems I had been blocking with tranquilisers returned and my condition had worsened to include a long bout of heart palpitations and panic attacks. By this time I had my diagnosis and knew something about the condition that I was dealing with, but I spent most of this period in denial about my illness, pretending that it wasn't as bad as it seemed.

This meant that night time was the time when all the pressures I'd been holding onto in the day came out in force and blocked my sleep. I lay awake watching television and trying to forget about my problems that way. There was a time when I could only fall asleep whilst watching television or listening to music because I couldn't allow my mind to wander without it attacking me with harmful, stressful thoughts that robbed me of my sleep. My hypersensitivity was also so out of control that ticking clocks and cars driving past the window were enough to make me give up on getting any sleep at all. I was in danger of falling back into the cycle of stage one's daytime sleep and then needing to return to medication all over again.

I broke the cycle. Now, in my twenty-fifth year, I can safely say that I have mastered the sleep conundrum. I have set a regular routine of the hours at which I expect to fall asleep (somewhere between midnight and 1 a.m.) and the hour at which I usually wake up (around 9:30 a.m.). Forcing myself into this schedule wasn't easy, but it has paid off in the long run. I have learned relaxation mechanisms to promote an easy fall into sleep (such things include avoiding anything stressful or upsetting after a certain time in the evening and not doing difficult physical activities at night). I also try to avoid sleeping in the daytime unless pain and/or increased exertion make it absolutely unbearable to stay awake.

The amazing thing about these nasty sleep phases is that once you've broken the original habit, it's actually much easier to stick to the new, healthy regime. Once I'd had a couple of good nights where I managed to get to sleep without the TV on, I was able to have faith in myself that I could relax and sleep even on nights where it seemed more difficult. You only have to get over that hurdle once to start believing that you can do it every time, and that kind of self-belief can be a very powerful thing.

Weight Loss

or

'Not everyone can be a supermodel'

I am rather fat. I'm not huge. I wouldn't imagine people are going to start chasing me down the street with harpoons any time soon, nor would I say that my extra weight is giving me any additional problems on top of my condition. I have big legs and a sticky-out stomach but I know how to wear clothes that hide all that and tuck it in to make me look just about average. I wasn't always this way; I had a period of time where my digestive problems were so bad that I dropped about 30 pounds (not a recommended way to lose weight, by the way). I remember what it was like to be that skinny. It was nice that all the clothes I tried on fit me, but it wasn't so pleasant to have every meal I ate come back up ten minutes after I'd left the dinner table.

I used to put weight on and lose weight depending on how my illness affected me. Sometimes I was so exhausted that I ate absurd amounts of carbohydrates just to have the energy to function and then I ended up bloated like the blueberry girl from Charlie and the Chocolate Factory and holding an empty pizza box screaming 'Why did you do this to me? You were supposed to be my friend!' Other times a friend might call round at six in the evening and say 'What did you have for lunch today?' and I would stare back at them blankly, realising that I hadn't actually had anything to eat at all since I got up. These awful habits and the way I changed them are up for discussion in the next chapter, but for now it's time to focus on how overweight that lifestyle made me.

As a woman who has grown up in the world of media, magazines and fad diets, weight has always been an issue toying with the back of my mind. I'll be the first to admit that I grab my stomach sometimes and just wish for it to disappear. Perhaps it's this particular brand of desperation that makes women so much more inclined to believe in the supernatural than men, but that's an issue for a different book altogether. The point is this: I am subject to the same social pressures about how my body looks as every other twenty-something year old woman out there. But I have this little thing called M.E. too.

I read somewhere once that the recommended amount of exercise for a person with M.E. was no more than 6 minutes a day. A counsellor I took advice from told me to start using my treadmill again for 30 seconds at a time to help increase my activity. Neither of these pieces of advice are helpful to someone who wants to lose their excess flab. I'm pretty sure that 30 minutes a day would only barely start to shift my poundage, so being limited to 30 seconds of mild walking doesn't inspire you to believe that you can ever have the body you desire. I am a determined person, one that likes to set goals and achieve them. I like to think that, if I were normal and healthy, I could be one of those people who did an hour's run on their treadmill every day whilst reading a novel and baking a soufflé in some fabulous Wonder Woman style montage.

As you may have guessed, that's not my reality.

My reality is that I am not active enough to lose the calories that I gain even from eating my normal three small meals a day. I will gain weight simply by eating normal things, even if I stay away from the dangerous temptations of chocolate, biscuits and chips. My output doesn't match my intake because my body is taking those extra calories and desperately trying to use them to do innocuous things like breathing and keeping my body temperature from plummeting like a reptile's. If I want to do more than simply exist, I have to eat more than the bare minimum in order to do it. The choice for me has boiled down to two options:

Be overweight or be inert.

As I said, I'm rather fat. But it's keeping me active, keeping me pursuing my life goals and keeping me involved in the small social world that I can stand to be a part of. This time last year, I was still trying to diet and following various plans that might help me to 'eat right' so I could shift those pesky extra pounds. It wasn't that long ago that I came to the realisation that my health is far more important than a number on the bathroom scales.

So what if my clothes are a size bigger than I'd like them to be (okay, sometimes two sizes bigger...)? So what if I can rest my phone on my belly when I need to take a break from reading (actually quite a handy place to leave it when you don't have a table nearby)? So what if I don't look like some magazine for healthy people tells me I should look?

Balance is my buzz word on this issue. I can't afford to take too much of a 'Who cares' attitude – if I put on too much weight, my muscles and joints will suffer even more agony than they do now – but I can afford to step back, look at myself and say 'You know what, considering you have M.E., you're doing okay with your body'. Not everybody is blessed with the ability to get control of their weight, whether they're ill or not, so I've had to learn to accept my extra pounds as a product of giving myself the energy to pursue the important things in my life.

I'm no stick-thin supermodel. I never will be. But clearly that's not what I was put on this Earth to be. M.E. causes its sufferers to have a lot of deep-set insecurities about their bodies as it is without them having to feel like they need to conform to the societal laws of weight and beauty too. So I say kick off the shackles of the scales and be the shape that makes you feel healthy, not the shape that ticks a box in some random column of media expectations. Magazines aren't crowding at your door to snap you and point out your flaws, so don't be the one to point them out to yourself either.

K.C. FINN

Eating Habits

or

'Lack thereof'

Habit isn't something that the M.E. body deals well with. Routine-setting is seen by many treatment programmes to be a vital part of resetting the body on its road to recovery, but the unpredictable nature of M.E. tends to get in the way of any plans that you lay down for it to follow. As we've already seen, sleep is one such area where achieving regularity is a distant, but achievable dream. Food and drink is another domain where teaching yourself good habits is really the only way forward.

To most healthy people, food is just food. You can have nice food, naughty food for a treat or good food for a special occasion, but mostly you just eat because you're hungry or greedy. For me, food was a nightmare for a very long time. Food meant hideous digestive pains, followed by a massive spike in energy and then the inevitable crash that made me wish I'd never eaten anything in the first place. I went through a period where I ate less than one meal a day, sometimes going from the time I woke up until about 6 p.m. before I became hungry enough to eat. I found that if I didn't start my metabolism in the morning, then my body didn't call out for food until very late in the day.

Did I think I was being clever? Certainly not. I was just trying to avoid more pain because I couldn't cope with the pain I was already in. As you may have guessed, hardly eating anything only led to shedloads more pain and anguish. I had gotten myself into a horrible pattern that was worsening my condition and giving me even more aggravation than I was experiencing before. Bravo me.

But what do you when your body is telling you it simply doesn't want to eat?

I had to use my common sense, for starters. Food is energy. A lack of energy is the whole reason my body is so exhausted and pained in the first place. I used to make excuses like 'Oh, I don't seem to absorb the energy properly anyway, so why bother eating?' It took a serious overhaul and a massive reality check to get out of that way of thinking. Everyone else in the world eats regular meals, and I needed to do the same if I was ever going to stand a chance at getting control of my life again.

Finding the right food was the first step. I took advice from experienced people (i.e. not the wild plains of the internet) about some of the types of foods that have been known to benefit people with energy problems. Some of them didn't work in the slightest, but it didn't stop me trying them all. The key is to only try one change of food at a time, so you can see whether it really makes any difference. Then, if it does, you start building it into your diet from there on in.

For me, foods that are low on the glycaemic index are my best friends. Once I discovered slow-release carbohydrates I rebuilt my whole diet around them and that easy-to-do change transformed my life. I'm *not* saying that this is going to work for everyone with M.E., because different physiognomies will react differently to each of the food groups. What I *am* saying is that if I hadn't been open to trying a new form of diet, I never would have found a method that significantly increased my everyday energy, reduced my daytime sleeping to a minimum and left me feeling like I'd finally made a significant improvement to my health.

The type of food itself isn't the biggest change either: the main part comes from sticking to a routine long enough to know if it's paying off. Tiredness and frustration make healthy people give up on things without giving them a proper try, so if you live in a state of constant tiredness and frustration, changing your routine can seem like the worst thing in the world. What I had to admit to myself was that my routine, comfortable and convenient as it was, wasn't helping me to be healthier. If can you trust in the hope that some small changes can add up to form a bigger one eventually, then you have what it takes to stick to a new routine. It's also been brilliant for my self-esteem to be able to celebrate that I have made a personal change for the better.

They say that slow and steady wins the race. From

my perspective as an M.E. sufferer, I know I'm not going to win the race, but I do want to finish it and feel that I've done well. This is true for all areas of my life, from completing paperwork and manuscripts to spending a few vital minutes a day walking on my treadmill. I find that if I stick to my plans as much as my body will allow, then the end of each week looks a little bit more hopeful than the one before it. I'm not saying that there aren't massive setbacks that bring me down again, but having a routine to fall back on does reassure me that I have a coping mechanism set up to help me get back on my feet.

It's important not to be fooled into thinking that there are 'quick fixes' for M.E. that will cure symptoms outright. I've had plenty of non-sufferers (many in the medical profession) who have told me that one thing or another is 'the key' to success. As I hope the many sections of this book indicate, it's the small changes that you make to every single aspect of your life that add up to an overall feeling of recuperation and wellbeing. It has taken me a very long time to stop listening to the many voices around me and look inwards to judge for myself what genuinely helps me to cope with this awful condition. Now that I know what my inner voice is telling me, I don't intend to let anyone else drown it out.

Diagnosis

or

'It's all in your head, except for when it isn't'

Myself and doctors are not a good combination. I have been through scores of GPs, therapists, psychologists, specialists, hospital staff, nursing staff and other people in the medical profession in my pursuit of information and treatment for the things that are wrong with my body. Since the age of thirteen I have been buffeted from pillar to post in search of 'the right one': that magical medical being who has the answer to the eternal question: How can I be healthy again?

I don't recommend having a bad relationship with medical help; it really doesn't get you anywhere. Generally, I tended not to trust doctors and approached each new medical venture I was sent to endure with huge reservations about whether I would actually find anyone who could help me or not. It's part of my 'don't set yourself up for disappointment' self-preservation technique. It's a sad thing to admit that I have been let down by a lot of medical people in the last twelve years, but it's even sadder to think that it has made me disregard the rest of the world's physicians too. It's not a nice thing to give up hope and think that nobody out there can ever help you to get better.

I'll assume that most M.E. sufferers reading this book will possess or be in pursuit of a diagnosis already. If you happen to be reading this book because you're wondering if you might have M.E., then save yourself some time and get onto a doctor right now about it, because if you do have this condition diagnosis will take you a long time to get and you're virtually helpless in terms of recognition until you have one. It took me nine long years of confusion and countless medical professionals before I finally got the letter that I needed to obtain fair treatment at university and in the workplace because of my condition. The sooner you start grabbing for that declaration, the better.

The trouble for me was staying persistent until I could find the right doctor. Losing my faith in medical help as doctor after doctor let me down left me reluctant to even visit the medical centre any more, which slowed down my progress in finding the right person to help me. Eventually, I heard through a totally unrelated channel about a doctor in a different surgery to my own that was 'sympathetic' to potential M.E. cases and was willing to do tests to help patients towards a diagnosis. I still had to be persuaded rigorously for quite some time before I changed my surgery and got listed with her, but had I not done so I'm fairly certain I still wouldn't have my diagnosis now.

'Sympathetic' is a funny way to put it. Surely all

doctors ought to be sympathetic to any upsetting condition that someone might have? It's only after having been diagnosed with M.E. that I began to see why someone would choose to phrase it that way. To a lot of people (and indeed a lot of medical professionals) M.E. is a psychological disorder. Many people hold the theory that sufferers bring it on themselves by believing they have it in some twisted form of 'be careful what you wish for' hypochondria. Because there's no definitive test result that shows categorically that M.E. is present in a patient's body, it can't *possibly* be a real existing condition.

Now I'm no doctor. I can only tell you what I know.

But I know that I spent my pre-diagnosis years attending full time education and forcing myself to believe that nothing was wrong me, insisting that I would get better in time if I just pushed the 'silly' thought of chronic illness out of my brain. I spent those years pretending that I was fine in front of family and friends whilst I suffered inwardly from crippling agony and unexplained fatigue that made me feel weak and vastly different to my peers.

And I know that since I've been able to put a label to my condition and to understand how it affects my body; my mental health has hugely improved. If M.E. was all in my head, then I would be healthier now than I ever was before my diagnosis, yet even though I have my life in good working order and am free of depression, my physical state is still getting worse. I know that my pain, fatigue and hypersensitivity are extremely real, so real that

I wish the non-believers (especially the medical ones) could step into my shoes for a day and see what it is I have to manage with each minute that I'm awake.

In my life, I don't have time for people who aren't willing to believe in my condition just because they can't see a cast on my leg or a scar on my face. My struggle for a diagnosis has brought me face to face with enough misinformed, pig-ignorant people to last me a lifetime, so my advice to anyone still in this process is to get out if you find yourself facing the same thing. Diagnosis isn't about sympathy; it's about finding informed parties who genuinely care about their patients more than the cost of running tests. It's about finding people who will ask you what's wrong rather than just throwing prescriptions at you at random. And, most importantly for me, it's about finding someone you can trust who leaves you feeling free from stigma and judgement, someone who you know has a genuine desire to help you.

So I may still cringe at the thought of each new doctor I meet in my continuing quest for effective treatment, but now I attend my appointments with a small semblance of hope that wasn't present a few short years ago. The right people do exist out there to help me, and it's only by continuing to navigate the dense jungle of the medical world that I'll be able to discover them.

Your Support Network

or

'How to NOT treat your family and friends like dirt'

M.E. is an incredibly painful and frustrating condition, but for me the worst thing about it is that no-one can actually see what I have to deal with. If I was hobbling around with a cast on my shin or an arrow stuck in my eye (just by example), then at least people who saw me would have some clue as to the feelings I might have about what's happened to my body. As such, this invisible illness creates its own stigma by omission: people simply forget to care about your health because they think you look well.

My personal beef is with Get Well Soon cards.

I quite often receive Get Well Soon messages from people who think they are being compassionate by wishing me all the best. I don't blame them for it if I can help it; clearly they are ignorant to my condition and that can't be helped in a society where half the populace still thinks M.E. is made-up. Let me put it to you like this and see if I can help the Get Well epidemic come to an end: If I was run over by a steamroller today and you knew that same steamroller was going to come back next week and run me over again, would you wish me Get Well Soon? I think not; it would be totally redundant.

My family and friends don't understand this mentality: they think I should say thank you to people who wish me good health even though I'm not likely to ever get it. Perhaps it's just one of my cynical bugbears that I'll never be rid of, but I suspect there's more than one person out there reading this who has a similar set of depressing emotions when a Get Well Soon comes through their door. The point here is that this condition does something to you that only you know about and only you can feel. Unless you actually tell your family and friends what's going on in your body and mind, they have no way of understanding you (and therefore no way to help you).

Frustration at not being understood breeds resentment, a topic I know a lot about. I can resent chairs for having more functional legs than me. I can resent innocent toddlers for being able to laugh without it hurting their facial muscles. And I can certainly resent the local bus driver for not lowering the disability platform for me because I look like any other twenty-five-year-old when I struggle up the step to get on board. Resentment is an appropriate emotion to feel when you have M.E. and you should absolutely be allowed to vent your frustrations and get all that negativity out of your system.

But don't do it to the people you care about.

My family and friends suffered for a long time at

the hands of my wild mood swings and random tearful outbursts. When I hit a bad patch, they sometimes still do. Pent up feelings aren't something that I find I can deal with very well, but the one thing I'm actively trying to do now is to find appropriate ways to channel them that don't involve blaming my support system. It's not their fault, after all, it's the condition's fault. And it's my condition; therefore it's my responsibility to manage it.

All your friends and family have to go on is how you look, how you act and what you tell them about how you feel. Two of those factors are totally in your control, so even if you look calm and placid on the surface, suddenly snapping at every word your friend says is going to send that friend a horrible mixed message if they don't understand why you did it. For my part, my self-esteem tends to make me think that people won't want me to tell them how I'm feeling, that they'll be sick of me, sick of my illness, sick of hearing where my pain is and how it's affecting me. The flipside is, I'm sure they'd rather hear me explain all that than bottle it up all day and then explode at them for no reason later on.

So here's what I've decided on the issue of treating your support network well:

Communication is vital; keep an open dialogue going about your symptoms.

And (just as important): find another way to channel your negative emotions.

You may have noticed the tendency towards ranting in my Get Well Soon beef earlier on. I find the subject so poisonous that I could have written that paragraph in my own venom. My mother puts my Get Well Soon cards up on the bookcase when they arrive, thinking that they're nice things from thoughtful people. I take them down and stuff them behind the books. She doesn't try to replace the cards and I don't shout at her for putting them up in the first place. We have found a way around the subject without it causing either of us pain. And then I come to my computer and vent about the cards here instead.

Writing is a powerful tool for getting things out of your system, whether you choose to make your feelings public, as I have, or seclude them away in a diary that you might later destroy. Catching a friend or relative in a complaining mood is also a good opportunity to join in and get a few things off your chest. If I were stronger, I might have taken up some light boxing and filled a punch bag up with pictures of all the things I hate (mentally I still do this and it's somewhat satisfying). Whatever the case, find your own form of punch bag and work the negativity out of your system. It's all just chemicals in your brain that make you feel that way, after all, so any method that helps you restore balance is one you should stick to.

Most importantly, don't ever put the people who support you in the firing line. They get caught in enough of your crossfire without you actually taking aim at them too.

Relationships

or

'Don't touch me, I'm a cripple'

My last serious, long-term relationship failed because I have M.E. That sounds like I'm making excuses, I know, but allow me to elaborate awhile. That relationship covered the period in which I became diagnosed with M.E. and also the beginning of my sharpest drop in physical deterioration to date, so during the course of that partnership I went through a lot of different stages in trying to sustain a successful romantic relationship whilst also fighting the inevitable decline of my physical health. Not an easy thing to do, by anyone's standards, but I lasted a little shy of four years trying.

One of the stages I went through was 'Pretend that everything is fine and dandy'. This is the stage that I would never, ever recommend that you try, in relationships or indeed in any other stage of your life. Healthy people with relationship problems might sometimes be able to pretend their way out of a bad patch, but the big lesson I learned in my 'pretend' phases was that hiding your illness only makes it worse. I once held the belief that if I could be a 'normal' girlfriend (or at least, give the impression of acting like one), then my relationship would work out okay and I could deal with my illness privately instead.

That doesn't really work when a guy putting his arm around you feels like a lead weight across your shoulders.

Physical proximity to people hurts me. Even a kiss on the head causes pain if it's in the wrong spot. Friends and relatives who know me well hug me as though I'm made of fibreglass. So if you want to be in a romantic relationship with someone, you can't pretend that this kind of pain doesn't exist. All that happens when you do that is: a) you end up in horrible pain; b) you resent your partner for causing that pain; and c) your partner resents you for blaming them without even warning them that they might hurt you in the first place. It sounds extremely simple put down in words, but it's a lot harder to lose the 'pretend' attitude when the pressures of affection and a desire for physical intimacy are at play.

So this is the opposite stage: the 'Walking on eggshells' stage. This is the stage where your partner is afraid to do, say or suggest anything to you because they are afraid of hurting and/or upsetting you. In this stage you remain physically healthy, but emotionally there is distance in your relationship and a barrier that can be both awkward and soul-destroying when you know that you used to be so close to that special person in the past. You may believe that your partner is only staying in the relationship with you because they feel sorry for you. You may believe that your partner is only putting up with you until a better offer comes along.

And so the resentment kicks in once more. There's nothing worse for me than feeling like a burden to others. Romantic relationships are supposed to be fun, enjoyable and mutually fulfilling for both parties, so when you know that your partner is unfulfilled because of you, that's a hard thing not to get upset about. In this stage I started to resent not only my illness, but myself as a person because I felt I wasn't strong enough to overcome my problems in order to hold up my end of the relationship deal. Not a good move.

So we come to stage three: the 'This isn't really a relationship anymore' stage. I went back and forth between the other two stages for a long while before this became my norm, and what a sad norm it was to live through. I had gotten to the stage where I was physically inert, reclusive to the point of not leaving my home for more than a week at a time and only receiving visits from my partner 'when he had the time', which was, at first, about three times a week. Then once a week. Then we went a month without seeing each other.

You have to know when to quit with some things. M.E. had driven a wedge between us that I wasn't healthy or proactive enough to fix. My ex was certainly no psychiatrist, so there was no hope of him providing the solution as to how we were going to make it through my rapid decline. So we didn't make it. M.E. killed our relationship not because all relationships for M.E. sufferers are doomed, but because neither of us knew the right way to deal with what was happening to me at the time. I wasn't ready to deal with relationship stress on top of illness-related stress, so I cut my losses and got out of Dodge before things had a chance to get really ugly when all that resentment bubbled back up to the surface.

I suppose the thing you'd like to hear is that I'm in a really happy, healthy, functional relationship now and everything turned out rosy after all.

The truth is: I don't want another relationship for a very long time. That's not to say that I don't believe in love or finding the right person sometime in the future. But right now I know that another relationship in my current state of health would be nothing but another disaster waiting to happen. If I want to play my part in a happy partnership in the future, then I have to work on getting 'me' right first. I have to learn to balance my symptoms, emotions and pain management properly before I can even consider bringing someone new into my life, whether that person is just a friend or something more.

Relationships are tricky things to get right at the healthiest of times, but I think that having an illness like mine has taught me a valuable lesson that a lot of twenty-somethings don't really understand until they're much older. If you're not in full control of your life and you're not satisfied with yourself and your situation, then don't bring another person into the mix. Make a priority of being happy with you first.

Action Management

or

'Life is what happens when you've made other plans'

One of the core treatments recommended to me after 12 years of suffering was the organisational technique of Action Management (sometimes also called Pacing). For those of you who've never heard of this treatment, it's a method of organising your time in advance so that you can build appropriate rest and recuperation times into your day. The theory is: if you pace yourself, you don't 'burn out' from over-activity and spend the whole next day wrapped up in bed moaning that your body doesn't work. Or, in my case, throwing things at the ceiling and wailing until some unfortunate family member takes it upon themselves to come and bravely listen to me vent my frustrations.

Action Management relies on the skill of organisation. Organisation is a big thing in my life. As a writer, I spend most of my time thinking about deadlines, setting myself goals, writing to-do lists and generally murdering trees with all the paper I use to arrange my weekly work schedule. And I'm also usually a person that organisation works for: I make schedules and I stick to them. I get things done by the date they're due and, in the cases where I don't, I have a series of elaborate back-up plans ready to make sure everything still works out rosy (some people would call that obsessive neuroticism rather than organisational prowess, but hey, po-tay-to, po-tah-to right?). So you would think that a little thing like Action Management would be easy for me to accomplish.

Yeah, well...

The problem with the M.E. body is that it pretty much does what it wants to you at any given time. Those reading this who have suffered for years may well have decided that it's their body that dictates what they do and how they behave at different times of day. If you feel good, you get up and do stuff. If you don't feel good, you lie around and wait (albeit impatiently) until you feel better. So when you're suddenly introduced to an Action Management schedule, your body immediately says 'No, I don't feel like doing that right now'.

I see the whole scheduling thing as kind of like being on a diet. If you're dieting for the day and then you suddenly become tempted to step out of line and, say, eat a huge slice of cake, your next reaction might be 'Oh well, I've spoiled the diet for the day, so I'll just forget it now and start again tomorrow'. And then you eat the entire cake and spend the rest of the week feeling guilty about it. This is what happened to me with Action Management. If I stepped off the schedule and didn't rest or do things at the right time, I'd then just scratch the whole day through and decide to do whatever I wanted to instead. And then I suffered for it the next day. The automatic conclusion that you come to in this situation? Action Management doesn't work.

My new conclusion is as follows:

If a method's not working for you, check to see if you're doing something wrong (because you probably are).

Most ordinary people wouldn't be able to stick to a fully co-ordinated schedule of their lives every day, because the world around them doesn't generally appreciate that they have a schedule and it will frequently throw things into the mix to surprise them. The M.E. body works in much the same way. You plan to write that assignment at 2 p.m., but the brain fog kicks in at 1:30 and you know it's just not going to happen. You want to go out for a morning walk, but it's pouring down with rain and you know that getting your joints damp is going to result in being stuck in an armchair for the rest of the day. So how can you be expected to stick to a schedule amid all this chaos? Surely you should just do what your body dictates?

The answer is no.

My body is sick. It's a constant parade of mixed signals going off at random times and places. It can't be trusted to dictate my life. Action Management isn't about meticulously following a minute-by-minute schedule and expecting your body to just obey: it's about taking control of your life again in a way that suits your ambitions. I want more than anything to be in control of how my condition makes me feel and the theory behind Action Management is a great one, if you can get it working in the right way for you. The hard part is then deciding on what exactly is going to help you.

For me, it was small changes that made all the difference. Whilst writing this piece, for example, I have stopped and closed my eyes to take time to just breathe. It's not something I'd ever done or even thought to do prior to being exposed to Action Management, but it helps me clear my head and physically rest my eyes between stints on the computer. I don't need to write out a daily schedule to remind me to breathe; it's just something I tell myself to do when the physical and mental stress of typing creeps in. Stop. Breathe. Carry on if you can.

I have been able to make small changes in other areas too, such as remembering to take pain relief at regular intervals every day rather than leaving it too late and ending up in agony. I set a rough time of day when I should be taking my tablets and tell the people around me so that they can help me remember when to take them. I am never bang on time taking them, but I do take them a lot more often than I used to and it's certainly helping to prevent random agony.

I have also set myself a regular time to get up every morning and, most mornings, I can manage it. Even after just a few days of having a strict wake-up time, my body started waking me up just before the time so that I wasn't screaming at the alarm for interrupting my dreams. I realised when that happened that I suddenly had control of something I had been leaving up to my body's discretion for a long time prior to that day.

Small victories are everything in the fight against M.E.; every moment you can triumph over the condition is something to be celebrated, so just because you can't plan too far in advance doesn't mean you can't plan at all. Plan small and plan regularly, and eventually those little victories will start adding up.

Work

or

'Believe it or not, I do want a job'

I am currently unemployed and making a negligible sum from the occasional sale of a book. Writing is not a viable career choice for making steady income until you've been at it for about ten years and got yourself established with a truckload of volumes on the shelves. I know this. I don't write because I expect to make a fortune from it. I write because, having left both full and part-time work, there would be very little purpose to my life if I didn't have goals.

Work capability is a big problem for M.E. sufferers because our condition is both invisible and indeterminate. The fact that a large proportion of the medical community still believe that M.E. is made-up or purely psychological doesn't help us much either when the dreaded government assessment for work comes along. I can talk until I'm blue in the face about how difficult my life is and how much strain every physical task puts on my body, but to some people that's all it will ever be: just talk. In the world of work, most people aren't interested in what you have to say, they want to see what you can do.

Well here's a little secret that M.E. sufferers don't like to admit: we can do everything.

On our good days, we can climb stairs, we can carry things and we can perform a lot of physical tasks. Sometimes we can even dance and do physical things for fun. We have the capability to do most things that ordinary working folk can do, so we always pass the physical tests for flexibility and capability when we are assessed. But here's the flipside to that coin:

Just because we *can* doesn't mean we *should*.

I could go out today and do a seven hour teaching day like I used to when I first left university. I could get on the bus, commute for forty minutes, step into my old classroom and give it 110% energy to get a day's work done. There's a good reason why I don't. If I tried to do that kind of day in my current state of decline, I would spend most of the next week in bed with every type of pain you can imagine running through my system. I would suffer enormous headaches from the overstimulation of constant bright lights and conversation in the classroom atmosphere. I would be hobbling around with my walking stick after walking back and forth in front of the whiteboard all day. I wouldn't be fit to do that day's teaching again for at least a week, and every day that I spent over-exerting myself would set my M.E. recovery back by months because I'm not following the recommended limit on activity for any single day.

As I got more and more unwell, I left classroom-based teaching and moved into private tuition. I could set my own hours and earn the same money for less physical time working. It sounded like a great solution and, for a short while at least, it worked. But soon even the twice-daily jaunt out to teach for an hour or two was too painful to manage. I had run myself into the ground so much in the classroom that even having some rest between teaching sessions was nowhere near enough to keep my health intact. I started to cancel private sessions left, right and centre, realising eventually that that too would have to come to an end.

My work situation at the moment is bleak. In my current state I am only fit to work on computer-based projects from home where I can set my own schedule. I have yet to find a job that will allow me to do this. If I did, believe me I would be the first in line to take it and work hard to get myself out of the benefit system. I hate being beholden to the government for my living and I want to feel purposeful in my life and earn my own money that I'm free to enjoy. I wish every day that I was well enough to work in a nice little office somewhere and build up some proper savings instead of having to just get by on the bare minimum that I'm granted.

Some professional people consider M.E. to be an easy thing to fake, even suggesting that many people who claim to have this condition are only doing it so that they don't have to work. The comparison between having M.E.

and being lazy rears its ugly head once more. I had a very enlightening conversation with a counsellor once who said: "If you wanted to make up an illness to get off work, you certainly wouldn't pick M.E.: it's too horrible to pretend to live with." I think if people understand how awful and crippling M.E. really is, then they'll be inclined to agree.

I wouldn't make up an illness that saw me spend six days a week confined to my flat. I wouldn't make up an illness that meant I had to sleep for three hours after a trip to the cinema because of crushing headaches. I wouldn't make up an illness that meant having to avoid eating all of my favourite foods because they irritate my digestive system. I certainly wouldn't make up an illness that sees me sweating buckets and projective vomiting in public places because my system is out of control.

M.E. is an ugly illness. It does horrible things to your body. It would be so much easier to just pretend to have a bad back if I wanted to get on sickness benefit for a while. I don't want to be on a fixed income all my life and I do envisage a time when I can get my symptoms under control enough to find a nice job that I can cope with without ultimately sending myself down the road of total physical burnout again. In the meantime, the best thing I've discovered is collecting together a group of trusted professionals that I can count on to fight my corner, just in case the government suddenly thinks it's a good idea to send me out to tend bar until 4 a.m. every night of the week.

Medication

or

'The drugs don't work... or do they?'

In the last twelve years, I have taken a lot of different tablets, sprays, inhalers, drops and other potions to heal what ails me. Some of these medications were pre-diagnosis, suggestions made by doctors to treat the various symptoms of my illness as they popped up, rather than stopping to look at the fact that a whole condition was materialising before their very eyes. The first tablets I was ever given to take daily were a preventative treatment for migraine headaches when I was about fourteen. At twenty-five, I've just been told it's likely that my headaches have never been migraines, ever.

A lot of people with M.E. like to compare medications to find out if they should be asking for something new from their doctors to try. This is because, for the sufferers that I've known, whatever meds they're currently on are usually not working very well. They keep returning to the doctors and trying new things, waiting for that wonder drug that's going to help them feel like a healthy person again. One of my long-distance friends had gone so far up the pain ladder that she was on morphine, but then even that wore off and her doctors wouldn't allow her a higher dose. I started down that road myself too, taking various kinds of painkillers and nerve-relaxers, trying everything that was offered to ease the discomfort of living in constant pain.

Then one day, I just stopped taking them. The mix of medications in my body got me thinking: 'What if half of what I'm feeling is all side-effects? How do I know what my natural state is with so many chemicals running around in my system?' So I stopped my tablets and let my body regulate without them to see exactly what was going on. Horrible, daily symptoms such as heavy-headedness and lack of concentration faded almost instantly, followed by a lot of the crippling 'crashes' I was experiencing between tablet times, which it turned out were actually worse than the pain I was trying to block in the first place. By clearing out my system, I could then see which medications were really working for me and which were giving me additional problems that I could do without.

Trying things one at a time makes it so much easier to see whether they work or not. I have been able to stay on a relatively low and non-damaging level of pain relief for the last few years simply because I don't have loads of other drugs saturating my system. This low-level relief doesn't cure my pain, sometimes it doesn't even work at all, but for me it's far better than suffering some of the awful side-effects I'm prone to with the more powerful remedies on the pain relief ladder.

I have tried almost all of the recommended homeopathic remedies for M.E. too. They didn't work for me at all, but that doesn't mean that I regret trying them. If any kind of remedy works for me, medical or non, then I keep a record of that being a good medication to turn to when those particular symptoms arise and need treating. By keeping my system clean of powerful tablets, I can try anything new that comes along and see how it affects it. Learning to say no to your doctor is also a useful skill in this respect; my new mantra is as follows:

If you find something that works, stick to it.

If you can manage with the medication you're on, don't go looking for more powerful remedies that bring more side effects and more inherent risks. The last thing anybody with M.E. needs is to make their body work harder to sustain itself. I know that a week's course of steroids make me feel like Wonder Woman, but that doesn't mean that I should be looking to damage my system by asking for them every time I have a low-activity week.

Part of this medication-balancing process also comes from having accepted that fact that you are an ill person. A lot of 'new' sufferers with M.E. (anywhere from 6 months to 2 years adjusting) try to continue living a normal life with mantras like 'This illness won't change me' and 'I'm not going to let it affect how I live'. Sorry to be the bearer of bad news, but you probably won't have a choice in that matter. New sufferers that I've encountered are always the most likely to make the doctor's run every four weeks to try a new set of meds as they try to regain a healthy lifestyle. I've been there, failed at that path, then accepted my lot in life to be permanently ill.

It's not a pretty path to go down, because when you fail on such a colossal scale with medication, the path you tend to take after that process is the one where you avoid all doctors and all treatment at all cost. 'Doctors don't do anything to help me.' 'Medication doesn't work because there's not a cure for this horrible life I have to live.' I can hear my own bitter tone from years ago echoing in my ears as the old phrases come to mind. I spent about a decade clawing up the steep side of the medication mountain and then crashing down the other side when I realised there wasn't a magical remedy waiting for me at the top. It is my hope that this section of the book will enable some people to go around that mountain and save themselves a lot of hassle.

Accept that nobody has a cure for this condition yet. Accept that lifestyle adjustments have to be made in conjunction with medication for you to go on having a happy, functional life. Try new treatments with an open mind, but a level head. Build up a collection of remedies (and lifestyle choices) that work for you and stick by them. This illness is an extremely personal thing; there are no clean-cut solutions that will work for everyone, so your best course of action is to get proactive about finding the treatments that are right for you.

Exercise

or

'You've got to be kidding, right?'

When you live a life that's a constant stream of fatigue and pain, regular exercise isn't something that ranks high on the to-do list. Adults who suddenly come down with M.E. tend to notice that all the sporting, keep-fit and other exercise activities they used to be capable of are suddenly unavailable to them, making them feel as though their whole physical lives have to come to a sudden halt. Mine was a different story. Because I began suffering with the condition at the age of thirteen, my 'sporting life' as it were, had barely started, so it was a little harder to notice the sudden decline in physical ability amid the huge mix of other things going on when you're a pubescent teen.

Hindsight is a very annoying thing. Now that I look back on that time in my life, I can see the warning signs plain as day. In primary school I enjoyed most sporting games; I participated regularly in sports days, did indoor and outdoor P.E. activities with very little difficulty and enjoyed playing tennis with my dad outside of school. Then came year one of high school, wherein I found I was nowhere near as fit and capable as a lot of the other girls, but I still had the stamina to keep up with team sports. I remember winning an effort prize for hockey because I was determined to hold my own against the more sporty kids.

Somewhere along the way, everything gradually stopped. One minute I was enjoying dance lessons to a Beyoncé song, and the next, every physical movement hurt. And I don't mean that it ached a little: I mean that an hour's P.E. in the morning left me on the verge of tears all day as though I had run a marathon. At this age, girls are taken away for 'the special talk' that tells you about how your body's going to change and how things might feel different to how they used to, so naturally I went along with that concept and just hoped that the crippling pain and tiredness from exercise was a temporary phase.

As you may have guessed, it wasn't. As I got a little older, I got very bitter about the fact that I couldn't do what other kids could. I blamed myself for my ineptness and blamed the teachers for not recognising that I just couldn't be bent into the shapes that other kids could manage and then fly six feet into the air on a trampoline. Something had to be done. So, at the brave and admittedly foolish age of fourteen, I made a stand. I sat on every bench and side-line all around the school, arms folded and point blank refusing to participate. It's an interesting thing to see a teacher come up against a student with that kind of strength of character. To their credit, they punished me as much as they were allowed to for my crimes, but ultimately nobody ever stopped to ask what the real reason was behind my sudden change of heart.

When people refuse to do something that you ask of them, I suppose the natural human reaction is just to think they're being lazy, awkward or that they want to cause trouble for you. If having M.E. has taught me anything, it's to pause for a moment before you make that judgement and consider whether there could be a deeper reason at the heart of that moment. Do they have a phobia or a condition preventing them that they don't want to admit to you? Is there an emotional, personal or medical problem stopping them from engaging with you at that time? I think it's particularly pertinent to ask these questions in this confidence-obsessed society where everyone hides the things that they feel will make them look weak. If you happen to be reading this book because you're looking for signs that someone you know might have M.E., then I reward you for your curiosity.

So how does exercise work in a body that's been at a complete standstill for a very long time (in my case, about eleven years)? The key is another one of those old faithful sayings that seems to have lost its meaning in modern-day life:

A little bit goes a long way.

You can't just 'get fit' with a condition that

presents you with crippling tiredness every conscious minute of your life. In the past I'd tried to make sudden attempts to calorie-burn and lose the excess weight that my sickness-induced lifestyle was giving me: things like computer-game fitness programs, exercise DVDs and 20+ minute stints on my home treadmill because I felt like I wasn't using it often enough. The result? Agonising pain. Days spent in bed having totally overdone it. Worryingly regular heart palpitations. Wild adrenaline bursts that woke me in the middle of the night. An all-around failure to perform, just like my breakdown in high school.

At first I took this to mean that exercise wasn't for me, but fortunately I was steered in a better direction soon after. Through the help of some talented consultants and the support of family and friends, I have finally started to see that exercise in the M.E. body is a slow and steady climb back to relative fitness. By starting with tiny goals and working your way up, you can regain mobility, strengthening your muscles without causing yourself extra pain along the way. The two most important things to remember are as follows: Start really, *really* small, even if you think it's pointless, and try it for at least a week before you think about making a small increase to the amount that you're doing.

I use my treadmill every day now, even though it's only for a few minutes at a time. I started at 2 minutes a day (which for some would still be quite ambitious), and there were some days I had to break that down into 'one minute walking, five minutes sitting down, one minute walking' in order to achieve it. But I did achieve it without causing myself distress. It might not seem like much, but to me it's an extra 100 steps that I wouldn't have taken otherwise, and it's also one of the building blocks leading to my overall goal.

I'm currently up to five minutes a day, which is a struggle to maintain when the illness is at its worst, but I am determined to continue making progress so long as it doesn't harm my body. It's hard to know that I can't do the physical things that other people can do, but it soothes my pride a lot to know that I'm making little steps (literally) towards wellness and mobility every single day.

Relaxation

or

'It's okay to stop and breathe sometimes'

One of the current theories about M.E. is that people who tend to be over-achievers are more susceptible to developing the condition. As a child who was incredibly driven towards academic excellence and success, I can see how putting yourself under that kind of strain might lead you to become vulnerable to illness, but I don't believe that it's the actual reason why I am the way I am. I still have the mindset of an over-achiever now and I still manage to achieve absurd things, like writing 78,000 words of a novel in fifteen days, simply because I was 'really inspired'.

(A side note to that is that I suffered with horrific back and shoulder ache for a whole month after my little 'inspired' stint and, whilst it gave me a huge buzz of personal achievement, it's not something I plan on doing *ever* again.)

I have mentioned elsewhere in this book that I am a person who likes to feel purposeful. I like to be able to say I have done something with my day, whether it's reading a good book, writing a few thousand words or solving a problem that needs to be solved in the house. I like to set goals to work towards. I like to be organised and tick things off my numerous to-do lists every single day. M.E. gets in the way of that a lot, which often forces me to put more pressure on myself to achieve things if I've had to spend half a day lying in a dark, silent room to alleviate my pain and fatigue.

The subtitle for this section is a realisation I have only come to in recent months. It takes less than a minute for me to stop, close my eyes and take in five carefully controlled deep breaths. The time I spend doing this seems a lot longer than a minute, but my clock doesn't lie and I can carry on with any activity I am doing with very little delay after stopping to do those five breaths. It's okay to stop and just breathe; it's not going to ruin my whole work schedule. In fact, taking in the extra oxygen from my breathing method is actually beneficial to the stuff I'm trying to get done. Oxygen is brain fuel, after all.

Relaxation seems like a dirty word for people who are obsessive, neurotic or anxious (and it seems positively blasphemous to people like me who are all three of those things). Sitting down to do absolutely nothing fills me with a kind of dread, like the seconds of my life will just tick away whilst I'm sat there doing this 'relaxing' thing. To prove a point to you I'd like to add that I'm typing all this with my left hand whilst I drink a cup of tea because I can't even stand to leave a sentence unfinished when I'm thirsty. You might think that kind of practice leads to endless mistakes in my typing, but I've realised something rather poignant through doing that simple, obsessive little thing.

I type slower when I have only one hand to use. And I make fewer mistakes when things are slowed down. Relaxation techniques such as deep breathing and quiet reflection aren't designed to waste your precious time; they're supposed to slow the world right down and help you feel as though time is on your side, instead of putting you under pressure. When tasks are slowed down and less pressured, you can do them well, often a lot better than you would have if they'd been attempted in haste.

That's all well and good. It's sound advice that I try to tell myself every day. But that doesn't mean I always listen to it. I will always be a hothead when it comes to getting work done; I always have that urge to burst in and do everything in one fell swoop. I'm like a horse chomping at the bit whilst it waits to race. The only problem with having M.E. is this horse usually collapses after the first hurdle and then she doesn't make it to race's finish line at all. If only she could learn to run a little bit of the race at a time and stop for a latte or a TV show here and there along the way. She might not finish the race first, but she *will* finish it and that's the important thing.

So here's what I do to combat the obsessive and the logical sides to my personality: I combine them in the form of an achievement chart. It's kind of like a star chart that you might have to get your kids to do chores and compete against each other to see who can get the most stars for being helpful and well-behaved. The only difference is I'm competing against myself and the goal is actually to do fewer things, not more. I reward myself for activities that involve keeping still and being quiet, such as listening to music or audiobooks, reading, watching TV and – deep breath here – building Lego.

I will do anything that clears my mind of worries and helps me to forget about my condition and I have never found anything so soothing in my life as following the instructions to build ridiculously huge structures out of Lego bricks. It keeps kids quiet for the same reasons that it helps me: it's methodical, slow and it totally occupies your mind. Whatever activity you can find that helps you rest physically whilst also encouraging a good mental slow-down, go for it and do it regardless of whether people will laugh at you for it or not. Anything that helps you to keep a lid on what you're struggling with every day is no laughing matter, except for when you build a really cool Marvel Quinjet and lose Thor's wig so he has to ride on top of it bald for a while.

Relaxation is a dish best served personalised. It has taken me a long time to compile the things that help me to switch off this manic brain of mine, so now I make sure I take the time every day to include those things in my life and encourage my body and mind to take a break from all the stresses and worries that M.E. inevitably brings me.

Ambition

or

'Getting what you want without killing yourself to get it'

I'm not going to lie to you. If you have M.E. and your life's ambition is to represent your country and play Olympic handball, your odds don't look that promising right now. Some people get better from this awful condition and some people don't, so who knows, you might be on my television screen getting a gold medal in a couple of years' time. But for the moment let's assume that you're in the same situation as me. In the last two years I have taken a serious physical decline far greater than any other 'bad patch' I've ever had in a dozen years of suffering. It has changed my plans for the immediate future quite considerably.

I was going to continue training to become a more specialised English teacher. The final element of this training would have included a six week intensive training course for 30 hours per week in London, where I would have had to care for myself, commute, study and work all the same time. Two years ago I said it would be a stretch, but that I could suffer it for just six weeks to make my dreams come true. Today as I sit here, even one day of that course would cripple me for a month. I retracted my application for the course a few months ago after finally working through my denial and accepting that I am no longer fit enough to withstand it.

I took up fiction writing during this same two year period as a method to escape from my work life, which was increasingly becoming more and more unmanageable as I tried to conceal my deterioration from my employer. I have always been a writer; I have been writing novels as a hobby since I was ten years old, but for some reason something clicked with the particular book I was writing and I actually managed to finish the story. Speculatively at first, I self-published the book and entered the word of authorship as a further diversion from the pressures of everyday life.

They say when life shuts a door it opens a window. Writing was my window when I was forced to quit my job and give up a lot of my training. I don't by any means make a solid income from writing as yet, but I am now on the path to being able to look at working from home as a viable career choice whilst my period of physical health is at its all-time low. A friend remarked to me that it was 'fortunate' that my dream has always been to be a writer because it's turned out to be one of the few things I can still achieve even in my lowest moments. The truth is there are many things I've dreamed of doing which I now feel I might never accomplish and having only one thing left to cling to has both upsides and downsides. On the one hand, I am pleased to have a purpose to work towards that doesn't usually diminish my health but, on the other hand, laying all my hopes on one dream sets me up for emotional disaster when things look like they're going wrong.

But ambition is a powerful thing; it is a force that has driven me out of my darkest times and given me purpose when the rest of the world has left me feeling like it'd be better off without me. The trick is choosing projects that are going to leave you fulfilled no matter what their outcome is. Regardless of whether my books get good or bad reception, I have had to learn not to hang on the opinions of others to prove my worth. The fact of the matter is that I have written thousands of words, created entirely new characters, creatures and concepts that have brought joy to myself and to other people that have read about them. That is my achievement to be proud of, an impact that I can have on the world regardless of who I am and what illnesses or challenges I have to deal with in my life.

I've mentioned several times in this book that the little things add up. It's true too when I think about ambition. Small goals and small targets can achieve a greater purpose if you just keep going and keep moving towards them. This condition has a tendency to make me feel like a bleak and painful future has already been arranged for me; I'm sure I'm not the only one who feels totally helpless when they're left alone for their brain to cook up bad thoughts. Having ambitions and seeing them through proves to me that I still have a say in the way my life turns out, that I'm entitled to have dreams and wishes just like anyone else.

M.E. is all about limits. How much you can do with the energy you've got, how much you can eat, how much medication you can take, how much you can sleep. I believe that achieving your goals, whether they are great or small, makes you think about limits in a different way. Finishing a novel was something I never felt I'd have the energy or mental clarity to do. As I sit here now I have almost half a million written words under my belt and ten new books planned for the coming year. Finishing that very first project, even in times of extreme anguish and difficulty, showed me that I could still surprise myself and find a new strength when everything else was turning to weakness.

If you were to ask me whether I think all dreams can be achieved, I'd probably still say no. We're not all Olympians, after all. But if you can find a dream that suits who you are and you're willing to put everything you've got into making it happen, then I'd put money on it coming true. If chronic illness is a concrete prison, then ambition is a wrecking ball with 'freedom' written all over it, and I want to be in control of that wrecking ball for as long as I can.

Deterioration

or

'The tunnel at the end of the tunnel'

Certain weeks creep up on me and leave me in a puddle of tears and regrets. The week that's just gone by is a prime example, as I found myself immobilised by lower back pain, weak knees and shooting pains in my legs. In times gone by this sensation would have lasted three days, four at most, but to my horror I found that this bout of agony lasted seven full days. I can't say that I'm free of the residual pain from it even now. This is a sign that my body is getting weaker and taking longer to recover from strain. This is a sign that my condition is getting worse.

There's a theory that suggests that the longer you have M.E., the longer you will continue to have M.E. Most people, according to the faceless research of recent times, recover from this condition within seven years of its onset. After the seven year mark, the percentage chance you have of recovering slowly decreases. I am now at the twelve year mark, which (depending on who and what you read) leaves me with about a 5% chance of getting better. Once you hit the big 20 years of suffering, it's pretty much a given that you'll have it for the rest of your life.

I'm gunning for that 20 line. Some people would see it as a negative thing to simply assume that you're never going to get rid of such an awful condition, but hear me out. I spent a long time going to bed every night, wishing that tomorrow would be the day when I'd just wake up and feel better. Every morning that I woke up in pain and discomfort left me disappointed that nothing had improved. Since then my gradual (and sometimes not-so-gradual) periods of deterioration have taught me that wishing to feel better leads to an existence of perpetual disappointment which is a terrible, soul-crushing thing.

So I see it this way. Let's assume that I'm always going to have M.E. and that I'm going to be stuck with its pain and fatigue my whole life long. There are two avenues open to me if I accept this statement. Option One is to collapse into a pit of despair, bemoan my unfair lot in life and wither away to nonexistence. Option Two is to take this knowledge as an opportunity to plan my future appropriately. If you keep wishing that tomorrow is the day you'll be suddenly, magically better, then you never take time to address the problems you're having today. How can anyone expect to improve their situation if they're just living in hope and not actually taking any action to change things for themselves?

I would be lying if I said that I don't take a jog down the Option One avenue when faced with the prospect of spending the rest of my life in agony. There are dreams that I have had to put away and accept that I'm not likely to ever achieve. There are times when I sink into the blackness of sleep and wish to some unknown power that I could wake up in someone else's body and let my own reality fade, as if it were just one long nightmare that's finally over. This last week I have contemplated ending my university courses, my writing career and my social relationships because I felt that I was just too exhausted to live my life any more. It's frighteningly easy to give in to the temptation of giving up on everything.

What I realised is that giving things up doesn't make you feel any more free. I can give up my job, I can give up my hopes and aspirations and I can give up people in my life who cause me stress and hassle. But I can't give up M.E.; I can't shake off that one core thing that plagues me day in and day out. The irony is those other things I'm trying to cut out to make my life easier are actually the things that bring me purpose and achievement even through my disablement. Persevering with the difficult things and seeing them through to the end reminds me that deterioration doesn't mean my life has to come to a total halt. Life can still continue and I can still achieve a lot, though I admit it's hard sometimes to maintain the will to keep on trying.

So here's where Option Two comes in: forward planning. It doesn't do any good to sit around waiting for the pain to go away and achieving nothing in between. The whole nature of M.E. is sporadic: it changes all the time, so one minute you could be in total agony and the next you could be quite capable of that walk in the park you wanted to do. If I'm in pain and can't do the things I want to do, I have to find something else that's achievable and work on that, however small an achievement it may be.

This is not always easy when you live in a world of ever-encroaching work deadlines, but I have to face facts: if I am in too much pain to get my work done, it's not going to get done. End of. So why am I wasting time worrying about it? If I can find something else to soothe my symptoms and occupy my time, then perhaps the pain will pass with less aggravation and less of what I like to call the 'aftershock' of a painful bout (which is kind of like the last couple of days after you have the flu: you're almost better but you don't feel quite right and things are more difficult to do than they should be).

Having M.E. means that I have a very limited time period in which to get my work done, but it also means that I have a limited time period in which to do things I enjoy. If my continual deterioration means that I'm going to have even less time for these things, then it makes sense to prioritise what's really important and what will bring the most joy to my life, and focus hard on that. If you can't see a light at the end of the tunnel, then perhaps it's time to make one of your own.

Raising Awareness

or

'The world just doesn't get me'

There were two things I had in mind when I began writing this book. First and foremost, I thought that finally being candid with myself and writing down exactly how I feel about my illness might help me to come to terms with some of the aspects about it that still upset me. The process has actually surprised me a great deal, because whenever something negative has made it onto the page I have immediately had the desire to counteract it, reminding myself of all the positive thought strategies that I have employed over the last few years to come to terms with my illness on an emotional level. In this respect I feel I have been very successful in exorcising my demons and putting them to some use.

The second consideration is something that I hope will come after this writing stage: the notion that this book might raise some awareness about M.E., C.F.S, Fibromyalgia and their related conditions in the wider world. Because a lot of books about M.E. are self-help books, only people who have the condition tend to read them. Their advice and medical guidelines don't apply to other people, so they have no need to pick such volumes up. This book was written with a very different intention in mind: to educate anyone and everyone about living with a chronic and invisible illness.

There was a sketch in one of my favourite comedy shows about three actors portraying different disabilities as an improvisation exercise. One actor wore a blindfold as he walked down the street, one was being pushed in a wheelchair and one looked perfectly ordinary. When asked 'What's wrong with you then?' the ordinary man replied (in an extremely glib tone) 'I've got M.E., I'm really tired'. Canned applause followed.

This show was made nearly fifteen years ago, so I can forgive the level of ignorance about the condition back then. What actually bothers me about the joke is that people would probably still laugh at it now, simply because they aren't informed enough about M.E. to know that they shouldn't be laughing. You wouldn't laugh about amputation, cerebral palsy or cancer, because you know how harrowing and awful those conditions can be for the people who have to deal with them. Plenty of media attention is given to these subjects to make sure you know they're no laughing matter. Invisible disabilities don't get the same treatment, even though they should.

Just because I *look* healthy doesn't mean I *am* healthy.

Unless you're also a young person with M.E., you probably wouldn't believe the number of dirty looks I get from people for sitting in the disabled access seats at the front of the bus. A fair number of elderly ladies with shopping bags have sat behind me and openly talked about how *disgusting* it is that I should take a disabled seat at my age. That's the word they use most often: *disgusting*. I'm *disgusting* for sitting in a disabled seat. Even though I am actually disabled.

Of course, when I get up to alight the bus and stumble forward on trembling legs, my face immediately flushed like a beetroot because my blood pressure has soared from the exertion, a lot of them regret their choice of word rather quickly. I get a cruel kind of satisfaction from having to rush off a bus to vomit in a public bin (from dizziness and blood pressure issues), simply because I know those people who judged me will be able to see at last that there's a reason I was sitting in that seat in the first place. It's a sad reality when you gain pleasure from something like that, but I did warn you at the start that this book wasn't all pretty.

Some people out there are real diamonds; they are extremely considerate souls who try to understand my condition. I measure my truest friends by those who have taken it upon themselves to read up on my illness and be aware of my needs without having to pry or ask me awkward questions; they surprise me often by being more well-informed than I am on some topics. But these gems are few and far between: the world in general is a media-fuelled place which only judges conditions to be important if they see adverts on TV all the time from charities asking for money to support them.

M.E. research is poorly funded and the campaigns that call for awareness to be raised are disproportionate to the vast numbers of people suffering with this illness in the UK and abroad. There are not enough people trying to help this cause and that's not because people don't care about others who are suffering. It's because they don't understand the kind of hardships we face, so they don't know how best to help us and they don't realise how little help our charities are getting. The condition is also barely recognised by the government here in the UK, making it difficult for people who are in constant physical agony to even supplement their income by claiming aid that they are perfectly entitled to.

My hope is that this book will join the ranks of others like it in a collective effort to lift the shroud of ignorance and misinformation that surrounds M.E. By reading it, people can learn to empathise with sufferers and the issues that we face. By telling others about it, the profile and awareness of the condition can be continually raised. All the right information on M.E. is waiting with the click of a button online, all those charities are out there who need fundraisers and donations to keep research alive, in the hope that one day there will be definitive diagnostic testing and maybe even a cure for this awful curse that attacks our bodies.

I sincerely believe that if people know about what

we're going through, then it won't just benefit us by the way they treat us in the outside world; it will give them the opportunity to help an underrated cause that truly needs more support.

Conclusion

or

'It's time to stop reading and start living'

This book has been a trial by fire for the last three months of my life. I have given up on completing it several times and even moved it into a hidden folder on my computer so that I could pretend it wasn't there waiting for some of the more painful topics to be discussed. Now as I sit at the end of this emotional road looking back, I find I'm very pleased with the result. I hope that these pages have given an accurate insight into what life with M.E. is really like, as well as pointing those who need help in some new directions that they may not have realised were possible before.

Drawing conclusions on such a varied subject initially seemed like a daunting task, but for many of the areas I have discussed in the book, the lessons I learned from my experiences were strikingly similar. Here I attempt to collect the key principles on which my life is now based, the principles which help me continue to strive for a healthier tomorrow and retain my strength in times when life gets difficult. These are my crutches, my shoulders to lean on when I need reminding of my life' journey so far:

Acceptance.

It is important to accept myself as a person with an illness. I am not like other people, but that's okay. I may have to do things differently, but I can still achieve what I want to in life, so long as I plan to do it my own way. It is important for others to accept that my experiences and way of life are different from theirs. They may not be able to understand what I'm going through, but so long as they accept me, they are worthy of my time, energy and gratitude.

Balance.

If my life is not in balance, then coping with my illness will be much more difficult. I have to make a conscious effort to keep my life in balance, even when that seems hard to do. This includes taking it easy when I'm very ill, but also not over-exerting myself when I'm well so I don't tip the scale in the wrong direction. I have to make compromises in my life, but they will be worth it if it means I can work towards a healthier future. Things which throw my energy levels out of balance need to be reworked or removed so that they don't set me back.

Patience.

A little bit goes a very long way. If I can introduce small changes to my life and stick to them, then I will eventually see significant and positive results. I can't just expect to suddenly feel better, but I can rest assured that

I'm doing my best to improve my life, bit by bit. I am in this for the long haul and my goal is to live a fulfilling life despite the obstacles in my way. I should always be thinking of the short term goals that I'm achieving instead of wishing for the long term success to hurry up and get here. I must remember to look back on how far my achievements have taken me so far and appreciate all the small steps that led to their completion. I can cope and I can thrive if I keep trying and keep going.

Consideration.

The condition is my enemy, but I cannot attack it. Instead it makes me feel like I want to attack the people around me because I need to let my feelings out. This is not the way to treat the people who care about me. Tempting as it might feel to act otherwise, I have to find proper outlets for my emotions and practise keeping them under control. This will not always be possible and I should always apologise for the moments when those emotions have bad consequences for the people that love me.

Strength.

Anyone who walked a mile in my shoes would know how hard it is to live with this condition. Just because the illness makes my body feel weak, it doesn't mean that I am any less of a person. I can take pride in the moments when I manage my illness and I can learn from the dark times when I find it hard to cope. I must be strong, otherwise I would have fallen apart a long time ago. I have lasted this long and I have achieved so much, there's nothing to stop me carrying on that strength and achieving more as life goes on.

Hope.

The more opportunities I give myself, the more potential there will be for hope. If I try new things and meet new people, new avenues towards good health may appear for me, as they have done in the past. Every improvement that I make to my life gives me hope that more improvements can be found. Whilst there will be many setbacks and unaccepting people that I have to face, somewhere in that journey I will continue to find the people and places that can offer me valuable guidance to make the rest of my life as healthy and happy as it can possibly be.

Realism.

I may never get better. I may always have this condition. I may, at some times in my life, be a lot worse off than I am right now. All of this is okay so long as I am prepared for it. If I can train myself to manage all the awful things that this illness throws at me right now, then whatever comes in the future will be no great shock. I will be ready to take on the twists and turns because I will find and utilise all the tools that I can to help me be capable and strong. Whatever hand life deals me, I will cope with it. Not just that, but I will overcome it and I will continue achieving and appreciating all of the things that are important to me along the way.

I said at the opening of this book that my writings came from a place of hope. At its conclusion, I pass that hope to every reader, M.E. sufferer or not, along with my wishes that something somewhere in these words will make a small positive impact on your lives. I know that in writing it, my life has changed for the better and I hope that in reading it, yours does too.

ABOUT THE AUTHOR

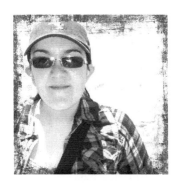

Born in South Wales to Raymond and Jennifer Finn, Kimberley Charlotte Elisabeth Finn (known to readers as K.C., otherwise it'd be too much of a mouthful) was one of those corny little kids who always wanted to be a writer. She was also incredibly stubborn, and so she finally achieved that dream in 2013 with the release of the *Caecilius Rex* saga, the time travel adventure *The Secret Star* and her urban fantasy epic *The Book Of Shade*. K.C. has also been welcomed into the fold at Clean Teen Publishing as a debut Young Adult author for 2014 with her epic Paranormal/Historical Adventure series *Synsk*.

As a sufferer with the medical condition M.E./C.F.S., Kim devotes her time to writing novels and studying for an MA in Education and Linguistics. She can be contacted about her work at her official website: http://www.kcfinn.com

Printed in Great Britain
by Amazon